Action Learning in Health, Social and Community Care

Action Learning in Health, Social and Community Care

Principles, Practices and Resources

John Edmonstone

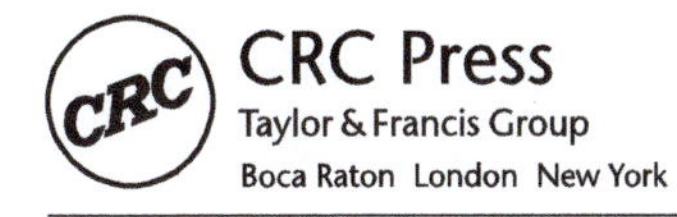

CRC Press is an imprint of the
Taylor & Francis Group, an **informa** business

CRC Press
Taylor & Francis Group
6000 Broken Sound Parkway NW, Suite 300
Boca Raton, FL 33487-2742

Printed by CPI on sustainably sourced paper

International Standard Book Number-13: 978-1-138-03559-1 (Paperback)

Library of Congress Cataloging-in-Publication Data

Name: Edmonstone, John, author.
Title: Action learning in health, social and community care / John Edmonstone,
Director, MTDS Consultancy, Honorary Senior Research Fellow,
School of Public Policy & Professional Practice, Keele University, UK.
Description: Boca Raton, FL : CRC Press, Taylor & Francis Group, [2018] | Includes
bibliographical references and index.
Identifiers: LCCN 2017016740| ISBN 9781138035591 (paperback : alk. paper) |
ISBN 9781138099579 (hardback : alk. paper) | ISBN 9781315266701 (ebook : alk. paper)
Subjects: LCSH: Health services administration. | Learning.
Classification: LCC RA971 .E328 2018 | DDC 362.1--dc23
LC record available at https://lccn.loc.gov/2017016740

Visit the Taylor & Francis Web site at
http://www.taylorandfrancis.com

and the CRC Press Web site at
http://www.crcpress.com

Contents

Foreword

I am delighted to be invited to write a foreword for this new book by John Edmonstone. A copy of John's earlier book, *Action Learning in Healthcare: A Practical Handbook* (2011) sits proudly on the shelves of both my home and work offices, ready for me to return to whenever I need inspiration, information and/or resources. My personal involvement with action learning spans being a set member, a facilitator, and an evaluator, and as one of the founding members of the Revans Academy of Action Learning at Alliance Manchester Business School, I have had the opportunity to examine action learning PhDs and to organise a range of seminars and workshops on the subject. More than 13 years after my first encounter with action learning, as a tool for individual and organisational learning within the NHS, the subject still excites, intrigues and reassures me and I have found in John Edmonstone's work the support, challenge and reassurance that I need in my task of seeking to inspire, and support, students, facilitators and sceptics of action learning.

The title of John's new work *Action Learning in Health, Social and Community Care: Principles, Practices and Resources* aptly encapsulates how and why this text has evolved. Its expansion to include social and community care reflects the changing context of health care today and the new emphasis upon working across organisational and professional boundaries, with a call for new innovations in commissioning to support the integration of services and the introduction of new models of care, such as Vanguard sites, devolution and multi-speciality care providers, in order to enhance quality and to manage costs. This need for health, social and community care to work together brings with it new challenges, new anxieties and new uncertainties. Yet a context such as this also provides opportunities. The very nature of action learning allows it to foster connection across organisational and personal boundaries and to facilitate the space to think, to reflect, to question and thereby to learn. This book provides an opportune resource which can enable us to develop the knowledge, skills and capability to seize these opportunities. It will therefore provide an essential resource for educators, commissioners, managers, OD practitioners, action learning facilitators, set members and anyone with the desire to learn.

Part 1 of this book provides a thorough explanation and discussion of the underlying principles of action learning. This section begins with a useful exposition of action learning principles, deftly weaving both its theoretical underpinnings and its practice to provide a secure grounding in the subject for those new to action learning, those wishing to deepen their understanding or those who, like me, are constantly seeking new insights. While there are many excellent introductions to the subject of action learning, where this text differs is in its consideration of the type of learning required for the current and specific challenges of health, social and community care and in its exploration of how action learning might support both individuals and organisations in confronting these. Following on from this in-depth introduction, the author takes us on a journey to explore how action learning differs from other development approaches, providing some excellent insights into the nature of learning itself. There is both a complexity and simplicity to these insights, enabling them to simultaneously support and intrigue those seeking to learn and/or to facilitate the learning of others. With the context now set, the book moves on to consider action learning as an ethos and a method, providing a pertinent explanation of its values and ways in which action learning has evolved to keep up with the changing context. This includes a very informative description of two increasingly popular forms of action learning – critical and virtual action learning, what they mean and how they can be utilised. Part 1 concludes with a description of the benefits of action learning, supplemented with examples of its use within health, social and community care and a consideration of how it operates across a wide range of different contexts and cultures.

With a firm grounding in the principles, types and benefits of action learning provided by Part 1, Part 2 goes on to provide a guide to the practice of action learning, taking the reader through a life-history of the action learning process, from initial preparation, right through to endings and evaluation.

Action learning, as a process of questioning and challenge, can pose a threat to the status quo and anyone who faces some resultant trepidation at embarking on its use will find helpful the section on assessing whether the organisation and its culture are prepared, can provide reassurance and an antidote to possible learning casualties, thus enabling practitioners of action learning to *'rock the boat'* without being thrown out of it! This section also includes a comprehensive guide to the roles and responsibilities of the various stakeholders in action learning and an essential practical guide to its components. A very practical useful part of this section is the provision of practical tips and resources, such as where to meet, how often and for how long, how to get the set started and how to manage the process of the set.

A requisite skill in working within any set is the ability to work with a variety of unique individuals. A way of understanding the contribution of participants to the set's working is provided in Part 2, through the introduction of the 'energy investment model', a model devised by the author to explain the contribution of participant's personal energy and attitudes to the set's working. This model provides an excellent resource for understanding both enablers, and potential disablers, within the set and will prove of immense value to set members and facilitators alike.

The practical focus of Part 2 of the book continues with a comprehensive introduction to the key skills of action learning and includes, for example, skills of active listening, effective questioning, reflection and feedback. The important, yet often neglected, skills of supporting, recording and ending the action learning set are also included, along with a highly practical explanation of various appropriate diagnostics and support mechanisms and their pros and cons.

A constant attendant in work in health, social and community care is anxiety. Despite being rarely discussed in texts relating to action learning, it is a frequent 'participant' and can have a profound impact upon the success of any learning endeavour. Its inclusion within this text is very welcome therefore, providing the reader with an explanation of the possible causes and manifestations of anxiety, as well as a guide which will enable the action learning practitioner to use anxiety as a tool for learning and to prevent it from becoming a learning saboteur.

In addition to this useful guide to understanding and managing anxiety as part of the learning process – a skill essential for any action learning facilitator – this book provides a comprehensive guide to all of the skills and qualities required by facilitators. This guide, coupled with resources to support the facilitator's development, and the means to avoid potential pitfalls, will be of immense practical value to any current or would-be facilitator.

Another key component in Part 2 of the book is the guide to the challenging subject of enabling organisational learning. In his approach to this highly contested topic, John reviews aspects discussed earlier in the text, in addition to insights from some of the major writers in the field of action learning, thereby equipping the reader with the capacity to support organisational development and learning.

One of the aspects of this part of the book, which makes it so very valuable to anyone interested in action learning, is the author's commitment to subjects often avoided in considerations of action learning. Evaluation is one such elusive topic and so I was delighted to find a guide to this practice provided through a discussion of the challenges involved, and the presentation of useful questions to support the evaluation process. With this resource, readers will be able to provide the evidence for the value of action learning in practice.

This practical part of the book concludes with a postscript which discusses action learning as 'reflective activism', a stance which entails reflection, active engagement in the workplace and the constant review of personal and contextual values, assumptions and practice. In this part, as in earlier ones, the discussion is of use not only to those interested in action learning but to anyone interested in the topic of learning per se.

Following this section on the practice of action learning, Part 3 of the book provides an extended toolkit of resources, which together with the extensive bibliography and examples utilised throughout the text, are sufficient to provide anyone interested in action learning with the confidence to succeed in its implementation.

What I love about John's books is how the author's drive to make a positive difference to individuals, organisations and society, jumps off the page, touching the reader and igniting their belief in their own power to do the same. I would like to conclude with a passage from the author's postscript in which this is particularly potent:

> In the current times of increased inequality and insecurity in the larger society, there is a strong sense of powerlessness abroad – a belief that nothing can be done to change the situation which people find themselves in. Action learning is the antithesis of this belief....in that it helps people to take an active orientation towards life in general and to overcome this dominant tendency to think, feel and be passive towards the pressures of life, ... rather to embrace the opportunities and challenges of organisational and social change.

Dr Elaine Clark
Senior Lecturer in Action Learning and Healthcare Management
Programme Director, BSc Management/BSc Management Specialisms
Alliance Manchester Business School
University of Manchester

Who should read this book?

This book is intended for a very wide audience.

It should be relevant and useful, for example, to senior managers and professionals in health, social and community care organisations who are interested in the potential for using action learning for a variety of purposes, including leadership, management, staff and organisation development.

A second group comprises the people who will have the responsibility for commissioning, project managing, monitoring and evaluating the use of action learning in local programmes within their own organisations. They will most likely operate under a wide variety of titles, often (but not exclusively) under the human resources function.

A third target group are the facilitators of action learning sets, located either within or external to health, social and community care organisations. The intention is that they will find much in the book to take, use, modify and incorporate into their own practice.

Finally, potential and actual action learning set members should discover, within the book, ideas and material which should enhance their contribution to, and ensure a valuable pay-off from, their involvement in action learning sets.

Acknowledgements

Many thanks are due to three colleagues who, over the years, have stimulated my involvement in, and fascination with, action learning. They are Mike Pedler, Hazel Mackenzie and Jean Robson. The bi-annual international action learning conferences initiated by the journal *Action Learning: Research and Practice* have also provided major support and challenge to my own practice since 2008. Fellow facilitators and set members have provided me with huge and enabling insights over many years and my own family – Carol, Duncan, Kay, Rachel, Charles, Finlay, Alex and Madeleine have all continually been my 'comrades in adversity'.

Author

John Edmonstone is a leadership, management and organisation development consultant with extensive experience within the public services both within the UK and internationally. He has some 30 years' experience of successful consultancy work in the human resource management and organisation development fields in the United Kingdom National Health Service, and within local government, higher and further education in such areas as leadership and management development, coaching and mentoring, evaluation research, partnership working and team development.

He has worked regularly with action learning since meeting with Professor Reg Revans in the 1970s, largely with health care managers and clinical professionals, but also in multi-agency contexts, principally within the UK, but also in Ireland and Indonesia.

He runs a successful consultancy business based in Ripon, North Yorkshire and is Senior Research Fellow at the School of Social Science and Public Policy, Keele University; Research Fellow at the Institute for Global Health and Development, Queen Margaret University, Edinburgh and Associate at Skills for Health. He is on the editorial boards of the journals *Action Learning: Research and Practice, Leadership in Health Services* and the *International Journal of Healthcare.*

He is the author of the books *Action Learning in Health Care: A Practical Handbook* (2011) and *The Action Learner's Toolkit* (2003) and is author of many journal articles on action learning.

Introduction

The purpose of this book is to demonstrate how action learning is a highly useful and beneficial approach to both individual and organisational development in health, social and community care. Action learning is defined here as:

> a method of both individual and organisational development based upon small groups of colleagues meeting over time to tackle real problems or issues in order to get things done – reflecting and learning with and from their experience and from each other as they attempt to change things. (1)

Health care is considered as the maintenance or improvement of the physical and mental health of individuals and communities via the diagnosis, treatment and prevention of disease, illness or injury.

Social care is seen as the provision of social work, personal care, protection or social support services to children or adults in need or at risk, or adults with needs arising from illness, disability, old age or poverty.

Community care is defined as the longer-term care and support for people who are mentally ill, elderly or disabled and which is provided within the community, rather than in hospitals, and which enables individuals to live in both independence and dignity and to avoid social isolation. This description is an elastic one and can be taken to include, for example, some of the activities of hospices, prisons, the police and clergy, as well as the independent, charitable and voluntary sectors.

While some of these services are delivered by 'statutory' agencies (particularly the National Health Service and local authorities), others are delivered by the independent, charitable and voluntary sectors. In practice the boundaries between these different areas have been, and continue to be, blurred and the need for collaboration, partnership working and even, in some instances, organisational merger, particularly between statutory agencies, has been increasingly emphasised over many years.

Whatever the nature of these organisations, one major difference between them and industrial and commercial organisations located in the private sector is that in the latter case there is what has been termed the 'reconciling function' of profit (2). In the services, which are the focus of this book, there is typically no such reconciler, especially since they are always part of a much wider system. The business of these organisations is therefore not primarily to make money, but instead to make a practical difference in terms of social change and improvement.

The book is divided into three parts. Part 1 addresses the underlying principles of action learning as both ethos and method and examines how it differs from more traditional learning and from other developmental approaches. It also considers the application of action learning in both business contexts and in health, social and community settings, with an emphasis on the benefits from its use. Part 2 explains the practice of action learning from preparation to evaluation with consideration of the facilitator's role especially emphasised. Part 3 is a compendium of resources which might be used by set members or by facilitators.

The book is both an expansion and a development of an earlier publication (3) but has been rewritten significantly in order to cover a much wider field and, in particular, to include material drawn from social and community care (4,5) as well as much useful material drawn from the journal *Action Learning: Research and Practice* and from other relevant publications, together with continuing action learning practice on the author's part.

Dotted throughout the book are a series of 'pithies' (6) – aphorisms which encapsulate complex notions in a simple but effective phrase. This was an approach favoured by Professor Reg Revans, the instigator of action learning, in many of his articles and books.

REFERENCES

1. J. Edmonstone, *The Action Learner's Toolkit* (Aldershot: Gower Publishing, 2003), 3.
2. C. Hampden-Turner, Foreword, in *Managing Public Services: Competition and Decentralisation*, eds. R. Common, N. Flynn and E. Mellon (Oxford: Butterworth-Heinemann, 1992), pp. viii–x.
3. J. Edmonstone, *Action Learning in Healthcare: A Practical Handbook* (London: Radcliffe Publishing, 2011).
4. C. Abbott and P. Taylor, *Action Learning in Social Work* (London: Sage, 2013).
5. C. Rigg and S. Richards, *Action Learning, Leadership and Organisational Development in Public Services* (Abingdon: Routledge, 2006).
6. D. Klein, *Every Time I Find The Meaning of Life They Change it: Wisdom of The Great Philosophers on How to Live* (London: Oneworld Publications, 2015).

PART 1

Principles

1

What is action learning and what is it for?

> The great end of life is not knowledge but action.
>
> *(T.H. Huxley)*

The working definition of action learning given in the Introduction to this book may seem to many people deceptively quite simple, yet it encompasses some very important ideas concerning both adult learning and organisational change that are significantly more complex and are central to what action learning is all about.

ADULT LEARNING

> You cannot teach a man anything, you can only help him find it within himself.
>
> *(Galileo Galilei)*

It has become increasingly clear that learning is an organismic or natural process, rather than one that is ego-driven (1). This means that it is not something necessarily which I purposively '*do*' but rather that it happens of itself, often despite what '*I*' want and not necessarily because of it. It is not confined only to formal and structured settings such as schools, colleges, universities or training centres, on educational programmes or on training courses, but is also informal in nature and so predominantly experiential, non-institutional and sometimes incidental – that is, it is often unintentional and a by-product of other activity (2).

As the theoretical physicist David Peat once wrote:

> Knowledge cannot be accumulated like money stored in a bank, rather it is an ongoing process better represented by the activity of coming-to-knowing than by a static noun. (3)

Therefore, there is no such thing as '*not learning*' because, in fact, we learn all the time, so learning is really continuous throughout our life. It takes place in all domains of human experience, and learning in one domain is therefore potentially transferable to others. The major issue is really whether the social and organisational contexts within which we operate either enable or disable our natural learning process. It is also clear that:

- ***Learning starts from not knowing***: It is only when people admit that they do not know how to proceed, that they are therefore '*stuck*' or '*lost*', that they then become open to learning. There are no experts in those situations where there are no '*right*' answers and no seemingly obvious ways forward. Where no right answers exist then people must act in order to learn. Action learning can therefore be seen as a practical means of sharing and exploring our ignorance and as acknowledging that we do not know which direction to take.
- ***Learning involves the whole person***: In practice, people do not separate their emotions from their intellect. It has been noted that:

  > Emotions play a central role in decision-making. The illusion that they can be somehow removed or put on ice whilst rational decision-making is in progress is neither helpful nor possible. Equally, the failure to manage feelings compromises the balance between thought, feeling and action. (4)

- ***People learn only when they want to do so***: People have an unlimited capacity to learn from their own experience, but a limited capacity to learn from being taught. Effective learning is therefore voluntary, self-directed and intentional. It is an active and learner-driven process, rather than a passive or teacher-driven one.
- ***People who take responsibility in a situation have the best chance of taking actions that will make a difference***: A belief in the capacity of people to make a difference in their lives is a key value embedded in action learning. Each individual needs to work out what really matters to them and what it is that they really want to do. This enables them to make choices and thus to take actions and then to learn from this.
- ***Much learning is episodic in nature***: Learning seems to take place in short bursts of relatively intense activity that absorb the learner's attention and is captured by the phrase '*I'm on a steep learning curve right now!*' The pace and intensity of learning then typically lessens when the immediate purpose has been achieved and at that point people resort to a much slower pace of learning before a further intensive episode takes place, stimulated by a further question, issue or challenge which demands resolution. This is because learning is a situated activity. What people learn, the pace at which they do so and the quality and depth of their understanding are all very much related to the circumstances in which they have to live and work.
- ***The urge to learn is stimulated by the difficulties we want to overcome***: The ultimate purpose of learning is to make a difference. People learn best from what they are doing, so real-life work and life challenges provide us with the best motivation to learn. We therefore learn best when applying new ideas or information to current problems and when exchanging feedback with others around practical applications. People who take responsibility in a situation have the best chance of taking actions that make a relevant difference. Learners can cope with difficulty and complexity from the outset, provided that they can see that such difficulty and complexity are directly relevant to their learning process.
- ***Learning is also about recognising what is already known***: Inevitably learning is based upon, and so builds upon, previous experience. It is not only the acquisition of yesterday's ideas but also includes trying out new and unfamiliar approaches. This means asking

useful questions in conditions of uncertainty and this, in turn, inevitably involves risk – the taking of actions which may or may not work.

- ***'Mind-sets' can be a powerful block to learning*:** These predisposing '*mental models*' or ways of seeing the world are the deeply held assumptions and generalisations formed over time by our previous experience, comprising our hopes, fears, dreams, speculations, queries, hunches, intuitions, habits, identifications, unconscious projections, half-baked notions, prior training, social conditioning and internalised social conditioning. Such mind-sets are usually not shared with others and are seldom explicit or even logical when viewed by those others; but they do influence how we make sense of the world and so contribute to the patterns that make some things possible and others not possible for each of us. They control, for example, how we believe that causes and effects are linked conceptually and they constrain what we see as being possible and impossible. It is important, therefore, that people need to recognise when their personal mind-set may no longer be valid, may now be less useful and so in need of review and revision in order to find new ways of doing things (5).

The difficulty lies not in new ideas, but in escaping from old ones which ramify into every corner of our minds.

(John Maynard Keynes)

- ***People learn best when they are able to question the fundamental assumptions on which their actions are based*:** Learning is increased when we are asked questions, or ask ourselves questions. Therefore, review and re-assessment of all experience – our knowledge and skills but also our self-image and our personal feelings – is necessary.
- ***Most people are open to learning when receiving helpful and accurate feedback from others whom they respect, value and trust*:** There is much that we can learn with and from other people that we cannot learn alone. Support and challenge from others who face similar problems in similar or different settings can serve to stimulate our own personal review process. It is much easier to recognise and to adapt your ideas when you have other people around you, facing similar problems, with whom you can talk. This is because learning is a social activity which is either helped or hindered by the framework of social relationships within which it occurs.
- ***Learning (and revision of mind-sets) is enabled in a safe and secure setting*:** Such a necessary setting is a means of containing people's anxieties regarding the likely impact of change on themselves and their organisations and of creating a space for them to work on new ways of tackling issues.
- ***Learning is 'amplified' when questions are posed and reflection takes place*:** Time and space in order to address issues, opportunities to take calculated risks, encouragement and support all encourage the process of reflection. Learning itself involves cycles of action and reflection. Working on '*out there*' problems in work settings also inevitably leads to learning in relation to our personal capacity and our emotional involvement. Working on '*in here*' issues of personal strengths and weaknesses leads to new experiences and to growth in organisational capability. The internal world of our thoughts and feelings and the external world of action and experience are therefore intertwined (6).
- ***The person with the problem, issue or question is the real expert*:** The individual with the problem is, and remains, responsible for that issue or concern. When they join the

action learning set they can expect to find help in addressing these matters but they cannot expect that anyone else will tell them what to do or will solve their problem for them. Unless a person comes to realise, on their own, exactly what their challenge is, there is little learning to be achieved by that person. The person with the problem is the only one who has access to the important information needed to answer the fundamental questions, such as '*Why is this issue important to me?*', '*What do I really feel about this situation?*' and so on.

- ***Learners need help and support (time and an enabling structure) to help develop their learning beyond the most immediate and particular***: Most people tend to look for early and practical learning that they can apply relatively quickly, rather than in the distant future. So there is relatively little interest in learning general principles. Once an immediate problem has been resolved, the tendency is to '*store*' how to cope with that specific situation, rather than to generate longer-term and more generic learning from it. Therefore, time (in periods of up to 12 months), support and challenge are necessary in order to foster that deeper and longer-term learning.
- ***All learning involves personal transformation***: Learning opens up new possibilities within human relationships. Through learning people can transform their sense of who they are and of the possibilities in their lives. It can provide them with a deeply personal measure of how they themselves have changed.
- ***Individual learning is a visible social process and can lead to organisational change***:

> At any moment we are prisoners caught in the framework of our theories; our expectations; our past experiences; our language. But we are only prisoners in a .... sense: if we try we can break out of our framework at any time. Admittedly, we shall find ourselves again in a framework; but it will be a better and roomier one, and we can, at any moment, break out of it again.
>
> *(Arthur Koestler)*

As such, action learning therefore differs fundamentally from, and provides a creative alternative to, more traditional and conventional learning. The latter is typically marked by what has been called a ***vicious learning sequence***, as shown in Figure 1.1.

Traditional learning seeks to provide learners with generic knowledge and skills but then leaves the challenge of transferring that learning from the education or training context into the workplace to the learner themselves. Learners therefore regularly experience difficulties in applying such learning to their local work situations where there may be few rewards (and perhaps even penalties) for trying out something new or different. This is popularly known as the learning transfer problem. The result is that workplace action often tends to '*fizzle out*' – to come to a full stop.

Action learning provides instead a ***virtuous learning cycle***, as demonstrated in Figure 1.2. Here the learning is focused on improving organisational and/or personal effectiveness, with the result that both the organisation and the individual learner perceive it as both relevant and easier to apply. Personal and organisational pay-offs tend to increase their enthusiasm for learning in this way. Carl Rogers has suggested that:

> Anything that can be taught to another is relatively inconsequential and with little or no significant influence on behaviour. The only learning which significantly influences behaviour is self-discovered and self-appropriated learning. (7)

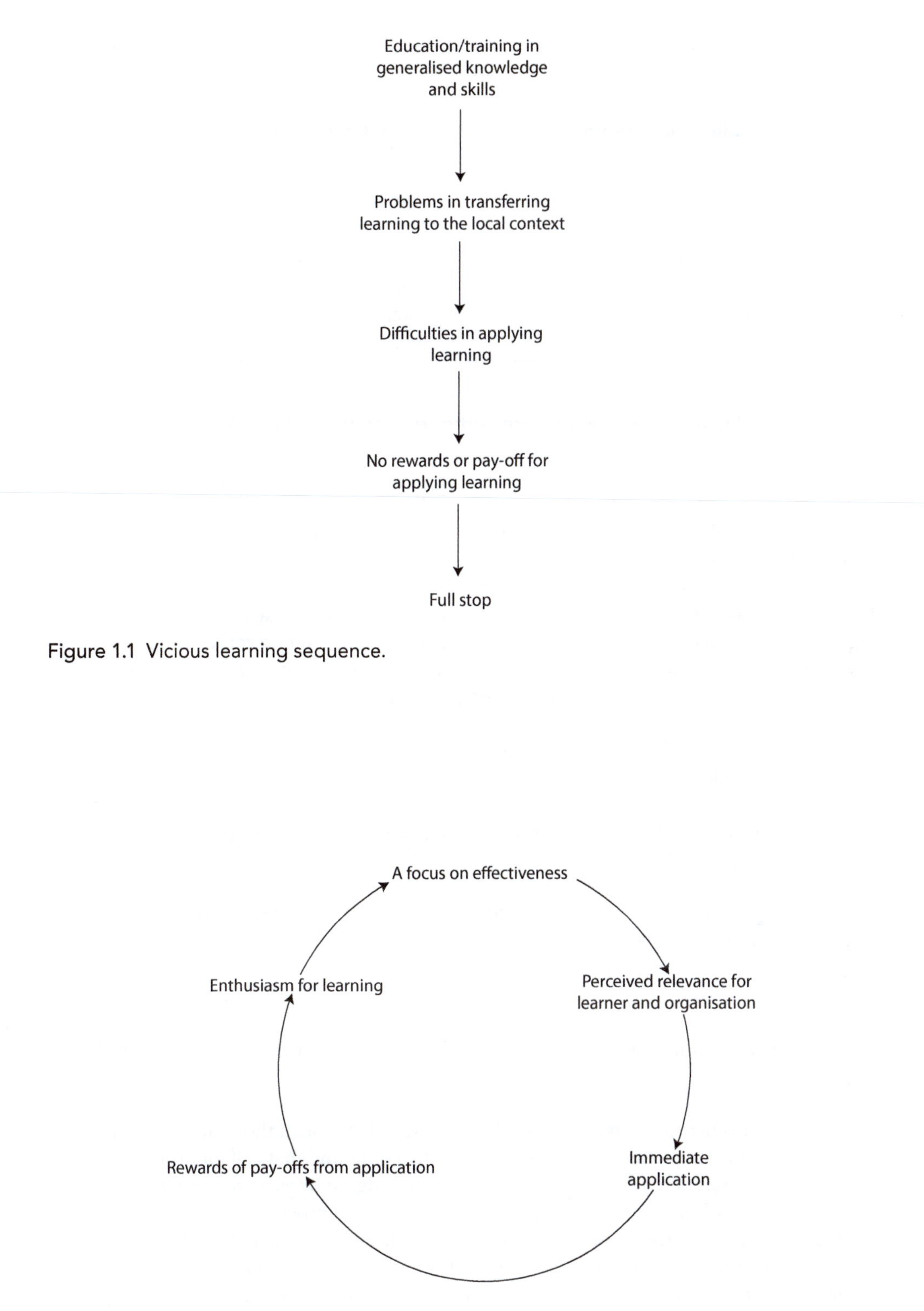

Figure 1.1 Vicious learning sequence.

Figure 1.2 Virtuous learning cycle.

The differences between action learning and traditional learning can be summarised as follows:

Traditional learning	Action learning
Individual-focused learning	Group-based learning
Learning about others	Learning about self and others
Input-based	Output/result-based
Past-orientated	Present/future-orientated
Passive	Active
Theoretical	Practical
Low risk	High risk

> Personally, I'm always ready to learn, although I do not always like being taught.
>
> *(Winston Churchill)*

Learners can therefore either adopt a surface or a deep approach to learning. In the ***surface approach*** (which is typical for much of traditional learning) the learner is simply trying to gather information one piece at a time and then to retain it for the short term in their memory. By contrast, in a ***deep approach***, the learner is intent on understanding an issue and with making connections between experience and new ideas. It is more long-term learning and comes from understanding and internalising something. It is therefore more '*real*' in the sense that it is less likely to be forgotten (8). It has been suggested that

> It is impossible to learn deeply when one is committed to being right in what one already knows. (9)

Surface learning equates to single-loop learning and deep learning equates to double-loop learning (see Chapter 3).

> A learning experience is one of those things that says "You know that thing you just did? Don't do that."
>
> *(Douglas Adams)*

Research on learning (10) has identified four distinct modes in terms of the way that learning is used.

- ***Replicative***: Where learning is prepared and packaged for use in those situations that are marked by the completion of routine and repetitive tasks and that call for little or no use of personal discretion. Here people learn simply in order to implement through being taught the '*right*' way to do things through given rules and procedures.
- ***Applicative***: Where the emphasis is much more on translating learning into specific prescriptions for action in a range of different situations. The emphasis here is on improvement and on working out how something that worked in one setting can then be applied in a different one.

- ***Interpretative***: Comprising both ***understanding*** (or ways of seeing things from a number of different perspectives) and ***judgement*** (practical wisdom made up of an overall sense of purpose, a feel for appropriateness and a flexibility based upon a wealth of personal experience).
- ***Associative***: Learning in a semi-conscious and intuitive way and often involving the use of metaphors and images (11).

Much traditional learning is concerned solely with Replicative and Applicative usage, but action learning potentially covers the entire range, with as much attention devoted to Interpretive and Associative learning as to the other modes. Interpretative and Associative learning involve learning to innovate through both critical reflection and the cultivation of effective working relationships with others.

Replicative and Applicative learning thus tend to focus on what has been termed ***explicit knowledge*** (12). This is what we can '*tell*'. It is knowledge codified into language and so communicable to others through documents, instructions, graphs, diagrams and indeed any medium that can be stored and transmitted. Explicit knowledge is what we learn through language and discourse (13). It is '*book learning*' – codified and recorded objective, rational and theoretical knowledge of universal truths, applicable not just in the '*here and now*' but also in the '*there and then*'.

Interpretative and Associative learning, by contrast, are concerned with ***tacit knowledge***, which is both personal and context-specific. Tacit knowledge is what we learn through our involvement with the world. It is subjective, bodily knowledge acquired by practical acquaintance. It includes our mental models – the paradigms, perspectives and beliefs that guide our actions – as well as our '*action knowledge*' – our skills, crafts and know-how. Crucially, it also includes our feelings, hopes, wishes, dreams and ambitions. Such learning is very hard to formalise and to communicate. It is probably far more extensive than explicit knowledge – what is expressed in words and numbers may, in fact, only be the tip of the iceberg. Tacit knowledge is the sum total of an individual's experience, fully internalised and more than they can express (14).

Action learning accepts the co-existence of both explicit and tacit knowledge. Explicit knowledge is the world of P (see Chapter 3) and there may be a continuous process of making some tacit knowledge into explicit knowledge through a series of '*raids on the inarticulate*' – of which this book is, of course, one example. These two modes of knowledge – tacit and explicit – are partners; that is, they interact with, and change into, each other as we work and learn. Once the tacit has been made explicit, we continue to build new tacit knowledge grounded in meaningful, purposeful and relevant experience (10).

This is not especially new. Aristotle distinguished between what he called **episteme** or '*knowing that*' – theoretical knowledge embodied in concepts and models – and **techne** or '*knowing how*' – pragmatic and context-dependent knowledge grounded in arts, crafts and skills (15). More recently, Alimo-Metcalfe and Alban-Metcalfe identified that the competence approach in education and training (see below) addressed '*learning that*' at the expense of learning with others or '*learning how*' (16).

The nature of tacit knowledge is captured in the joke about the man who came to repair a boiler that had ceased working. The man looked at the boiler for five minutes and then pulled out a hammer and tapped the boiler in a particular spot, at which point it roared back into life. When he was questioned about his £100 fee for repairing the boiler, the man said '*£5 is for my time, but £95 is for knowing where to tap the boiler!*' This is tacit knowledge or techne in action.

A number of common, but false, assumptions underlie the more traditional approach to learning. Specifically, they are that:

- Learning theory and doing things in practice are quite separate activities.
- Theory must be known before practice can be successfully attempted.
- Knowing the theory and performing '*routinely*' are all that is required.
- Learning and improving work practice are merely about repeating routines.
- What makes a person expert in their field is their theoretical knowledge.
- Such theoretical knowledge is itself absolute and unproblematic.
- Mastery of theory will ensure mastery of practice.
- Theory comes from research and investigation and it is the individual learner's responsibility to apply it unquestioningly to practice.

This leads to an over-concentration of much traditional education and training activity on technical (or explicit) knowledge and to the creation of a false dichotomy between that and practical (or tacit) knowledge (10), as shown in Figure 1.3.

It is perhaps not surprising to learn, therefore, that action learning may sometimes be difficult to implement in those national and organisational cultures that have historically been marked by largely didactic approaches to education and training (17).

This focus on technical or explicit knowledge is exemplified by the popularity of the competency-based approach to education and training. **Competence** has been defined as being concerned with what individuals know or are able to do, in terms of their knowledge, skills and attitudes. Competence works well with '*tame*' issues (18), where the issue concerned is clear and unambiguous and where tried and tested solutions can be applied. It suffices when there are high degrees of certainty and agreement and where the task to be done and the setting

Technical/explicit knowledge	**Practical/tacit knowledge**
Typically codified and written	Typically expressed in practice and learned only through experience
Based on established practice	Based on established practice modified by idiosyncratic technique
In accordance with prescription	Loosely, variably, uniquely. In a discretionary way based on personal insight
Used in clearly defined circumstances	Used in both expected and unexpected circumstances
To achieve an envisaged and familiar result	To achieve an indefinite or novel result
Emphasis on routine – method, analysis, planning	Emphasis on non-routine – variety, invention, responsiveness
Focus on well-defined problems	Focus on poorly defined problems

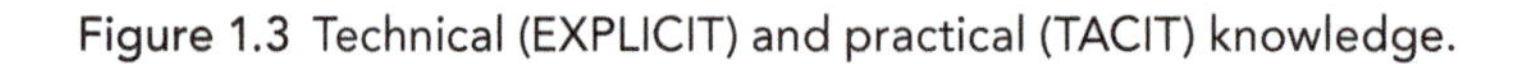

Figure 1.3 Technical (EXPLICIT) and practical (TACIT) knowledge.

in which it is to be accomplished are both familiar. However, increasingly individuals and organisations find themselves in situations where there is little certainty and agreement, where both task and setting are unfamiliar and where old and familiar solutions simply do not work. What is required here is **capability**, which is future-orientated and concerned with the extent to which individual learners can cope with uncertainty, can adapt to change, can generate new knowledge and can continue to improve their performance. It is therefore the fundamental basis from which an individual develops their own future competence.

Increasingly people have to cope on a regular basis with complex and uncertain situations where previously operated knowledge and preferred routines fall short or do not fit what is happening. In such cases, what works is not adherence to the previously known and trusted procedures, a pretence that surprise elements do not exist or an expansion of current procedures in order to '*nail down*' the problem. This relates to the growing recognition, derived from the development of professional practice, that people usually think and do at the same time (11) and that thinking and doing influence each other. We regulate what we do appropriately to the actual situation we find ourselves in – the setting or context that we are in inevitably shapes our reaction.

What might be termed '*intelligent performance*' – where people are thinking about what they are doing as they are doing it – exemplifies a movement to reflecting in practice (19) and does not depend upon previously learned rules. It is possible to '*do*' before the rules for doing are even known, as is demonstrated by small children who can balance on a bicycle without knowing the physics of the activity they are engaged in. We can perform intelligently long before we are able to articulate the principles of our performance. Theory and practice are inter-related and become one in practice. Practice often precedes theory and theorising is, in fact, a form of practice. Learning to '*do*' involves thinking, judgement, decision-making and improvisation. Simply repeating routines is unlikely to improve practice, but much more likely to produce automatons. To practice successfully therefore involves the development of capability, which comprises, for people working in health, social and community care:

- A primary concern for, and an understanding of, patients/clients/service users and their needs
- An ability to read and to analyse a particular situation and problem and to respond creatively to what is seen
- The ability to draw upon a number of different approaches and to discriminate between them, based upon the merits of each – a personal repertoire
- A willingness to continuously learn by experiment, reflection and review of experience
- A concern to work by trial and error – but systematically
- The ability to theorise about practice during practice – to turn instinct into insight by thinking about what one is doing as one works and arguing about it in one's head and with others
- From this, the ability to draw-out the theory underlying our actions
- The ability to relate emerging personal theory and practice to wider considerations of theory and practice: to self-evaluate practice in order to improve it
- A concern with knowledge in use and the creation of future knowledge
- An understanding of, and a concern with, the role of the profession or occupation in society (10)

This is just as true of leadership and management within health, social and community care organisations as it is for professional practice within those same organisations. Using the metaphor of performing art for the work of managerial leaders, for example, it has been suggested that:

> They learn their art by performing it. They discover new depths to the soliloquy, the cadenza, the pas-de-deux, by performing it. Yes, by reflecting on it; yes, by experimenting with it; yes, by repeating it over and over. But all these ways of learning presume that the performers are doing the activities in the first place. (20)

The challenge for health, social and community care organisations is to develop both competence **and** capability, but the key to survival and success lies more with the latter than with the former. A focus only on competence alone can produce good '*technicians*' who can work well at the Replicative and Applicative levels, but a concern for both competence and capability ensures the development of true professionals.

Action learning is thus a powerful and creative alternative to more traditional learning. The latter is typically marked by a prescribed, didactic, expert-based transmission of what worked yesterday, whereas action learning emphasises relevance, usefulness and a concern with what will work today and tomorrow. Some years ago it was noted that:

> Now we need people who can flex and adapt quickly, who develop complex and personal repertoires of skills and responses which enable them to get by and survive and prosper. People who can forget skills as quickly as they can learn them are more likely to be valued in a world where organisations are formed and dissolved in half a generation, rather than over generations of seemingly predictable progression. (21)

There are also a number of other important differences between action learning and traditional learning:

- Compared with traditional learning, the relationship between theory and practice is reversed in action learning. Theory is created through reflection and dialogue in order to explain and to clarify experience, rather than learned (supposedly completely) before experience is even attempted.
- This results in the lack of any defined '*curriculum*' or pre-determined specification of knowledge. This, in turn, of course, makes evaluation of action learning difficult because what is learned is not specified in advance or in any detail, if at all, and may not even always be what was originally intended (see Chapter 13).
- Action learning changes the power relationship in the learning situation. Neither the action learning set facilitator nor the set member's employing organisation is wholly in charge. Compared with more conventional and formal learning methods, accountability for what is learned remains largely with the individual learner.

> It is what we think we already know that prevents us from learning.
>
> *(Claude Bernard)*

ORGANISATIONAL CHANGE

The values, assumptions and beliefs underpinning action learning have much in common with the field of Organisation Development (OD) and there is a powerful case for considering them as overlapping fields of practice (22). The major text on OD (23) identifies a number of key underlying assumptions about how organisations work:

- ***The basic building-blocks of an organisation are groups*:** So the basic units of organisational change are also groups.
- ***The fostering of more collaborative working within and between organisations is important*:** So an important change goal is to reduce inappropriate conflict.
- ***Decision-making should be located where information sources are*:** Successful organisations tend not to operate in overly hierarchical ways.
- ***Continuous management against goals is central*:** For individuals, parts of organisations and whole organisations.
- ***More open communication, mutual trust and confidence is necessary*:** So a major goal of healthy organisations must be to foster this between different functions, professions and organisational levels.
- ***People support what they help to create*:** Those affected by a change need to have an active participation in that change and a sense of ownership in its planning and conduct.

These values can be summarised as trust and respect for the individual; legitimacy of feelings; open communication; decentralised decision-making; participation and contribution by all organisation members; collaboration and cooperation; appropriate use of power and authentic interpersonal relations. Taken together, these values, and the practices which flow from them, serve to enhance ***systemic eloquence*** – the ability of parts of a system – an organisation, a group of organisations or a network – to talk well to each other.

The most major evaluation of action learning ever conducted was of the Hospital Internal Communications (HIC) programme which focused on organisational change in health. It demonstrated that action learning was highly effective in bringing about such organisational change through individual change (24). A later review of action learning using the Return on Investment (ROI) approach concluded that, at an organisational level, it had achieved both significant cost-savings and also fostered revenue-raising initiatives (25).

There is, however, also an important difference between action learning and OD. Much of the theory and practice of OD adopts an ***outside-in process***:

- It starts with an emphasis on predetermined or given organisational imperatives and the requirements of specific organisational roles.
- From this it produces a projected '*ideal*' state of affairs and models or roles – often expressed in terms of competences.
- It then involves processes of appraisal and assessment against the ideal in order to identify the '*deficit*'.
- It then sees OD interventions as a means of filling the deficit or gap.

This approach reflects an ***extrinsic orientation*** and is essentially '*instrumentalist*' in nature – it sees action learning as merely a '*tool*' – a means of moving towards previously defined purposes (26).

The origins of OD lie in the mid-twentieth century United States, significantly through the notion of planned organisational change based upon behavioural science theory (especially social psychology) and consultancy practice. More recently it has become subject to increasing criticism as being, in its current form, less well-fitted to meet present and future organisational and social challenges (27,28).

By contrast, action learning embodies an ***inside-out process***, based on:

- A whole-person focus
- Seeing personal and organisational change as a '*journey, not a destination*' – as operating on the edge of possibility and enabling people to construct maps showing where they have come from, where they are now and where they might go in future
- Seeking to balance both support and challenge and action and reflection

This is reflective of an ***intrinsic orientation*** to learning, centred primarily on the individual and their learning, where learning is seen to be valuable in and of itself.

> People need to act in order to discover what they face; they need to talk in order to discover what they think and they need to feel in order to discover what it all means.
>
> *(Karl Weick)*

In contrast to OD, action learning originated in the UK, where Revans began as a scientist and moved through operational research towards applied science and problem-solving. His great insight was that a rational economic approach was insufficient and this led him towards considerations of adult learning. From the 1980s action learning graduated from Revans' original pioneering work in mines, factories, schools and hospitals to much wider applications in the development of people and organisations. This resurgence has accelerated internationally (see Chapter 4) and action learning is now established in the education and development mainstream in many organisations and sectors and in many countries.

From about the 1980s, action learning became increasingly individual focused, but when Revans evolved his ideas of action learning from the late 1940s to the 1970s it was already clear that there was an organisational, and indeed a societal focus too. Revans' work in Belgium, for example, was not just linked into organisational change but was also designed to make an impact on the Belgian economy (29).

Thus, with its roots in both adult learning and organisational change, action learning has three mutually reinforcing purposes:

- ***To make things happen***: To make useful progress on the treatment of a perplexing problem, issue, question or opportunity in the real world that had previously seemed insoluble, either within an organisation or between organisations.
- ***To help people learn how to learn***: Enabling individuals to deal with such problems or issues in the future, and so ensuring the transfer of learning from one situation or setting to others.
- ***To help build a learning organisation***: To foster an internal organisational learning '*architecture*' so that continuing learning and development are permanent features of organisational life, so helping individuals and organisations to survive and to prosper in a complex and confusing world.

THE TITANIC CONNECTION

Professor Reg Revans was the acknowledged '*father*' of action learning. An award-winning student of physics at Cambridge University in the 1930s, he also represented Great Britain at the Amsterdam Olympics of 1928. While at Cambridge, working under the supervision of Lord Rutherford, he developed his first original thinking on action learning and experienced first-hand the usefulness of team-working, collaborative thinking and the merits of having views challenged by co-workers.

However, although he was only a small boy at the time, the sinking of the Titanic in 1912 with over 1400 passengers had left a lasting legacy in Revans' ideas. Questions were raised on both sides of the Atlantic as to how such an allegedly unsinkable ship could have gone down on its maiden voyage. What had happened? What had gone wrong? Why could no-one have foreseen such an event? Revans' father was the Principal Surveyor of Mercantile Shipping and was deeply involved in the official inquiry into the sinking. Several of the designers and constructors of the vessel had, in fact, been concerned, but had never raised their concerns with their colleagues. They seemed to be afraid of appearing foolish by asking '*stupid*' questions. A procession of poverty-stricken sailors also came barefoot to the Revans' home to report on their experiences aboard the ill-fated liner and his father's accounts of this made a lasting impression on Revans. His father had heard, time and again, how the sailors had tried to warn those in authority about the risks posed by trying to break the transatlantic record and how these views had been ignored – with disastrous results. The lesson was not lost on Revans. The need to value all views, regardless of hierarchy or status, and the importance of distinguishing between '*cleverness*' and '*wisdom*' underpinned his ideas on action learning and his advocacy of egalitarian approaches as the basis for action learning sets.

> The concept of action learning teaches participants to act themselves into a new way of thinking, rather than think themselves into a new way of acting.
>
> *(Reg Revans)*

REFERENCES

1. G. Claxton, *Wholly Human: Western and Eastern Visions of the Self and Its Perfection* (London: Routledge & Kegan Paul, 1981).
2. V. Marsick and K. Watkins, Lessons from informal and incidental learning, in *Management Learning: Integrating Perspectives in Theory and Practice*, eds. John Burgoyne and Mike Reynolds (London: Sage, 1997).
3. D. Peat, *Blackfoot Physics* (London: Fourth Estate, 1996).
4. T. Morrison, Emotional intelligence, emotion and social work: Context, characteristics, complications and contribution, *British Journal of Social Work* 37 (2); 2007: 245–263.
5. M. Magzan, Mental models for leadership effectiveness: Building futures different than the past, *Journal of Engineering Management and Competitiveness* 2 (2); 2012: 57–63.
6. L. Beaty, *Action Learning* (York: Learning & Teaching Support Network CPD Paper 1, 2003).
7. C. Rogers, *On Becoming A Person* (Boston, MA: Houghton-Mifflin, 1961).
8. F. Marton and R. Saljo, On qualitative differences in learning: 1: Outcome and process, *British Journal of Educational Psychology* 46; 1976: 4–11.
9. I. Price and R. Shaw, *Shifting the Patterns: Breaking the Memetic Codes of Corporate Performance* (Chalford: Management Books 2000, 1998).
10. M. Eraut, *Developing Professional Knowledge and Competence* (London: Falmer Press, 1994).

11. G. Claxton, *Hare Brain: Tortoise Mind: Why Intelligence Increases When You Think Less* (London: Fourth Estate, 1997).
12. M. Polanyi, *The Tacit Dimension* (London: Routledge & Kegan Paul, 1966).
13. B. Garvey and B. Williamson, *Beyond Knowledge Management: Dialogue, Creativity and the Corporate Curriculum* (Harlow: Pearson Education/ Prentice-Hall, 2002).
14. I. Nonaka and H. Takeuchi, *The Knowledge-Creating Company: How Japanese Companies Create the Dynamics of Innovation* (Oxford: Oxford University Press, 1995).
15. Aristotle, *The Nicomachean Ethics* (London: Penguin, 2004).
16. B. Alimo-Metcalfe and J. Alban-Metcalfe, *Engaging Leadership: Creating Organisations that Maximise the Potential of Their People* (London: Chartered Institute of Personnel and Development, 2008).
17. A. Pun, Action learning: Encountering Chinese culture, in *Human Resource Development: International Perspectives on Development and Learning* eds. M. Jones and P. Mann (West Hartford, CT: Kumarian Press, 1992).
18. H. Rittel and M. Webber, Dilemmas in a general theory of planning, *Policy Science* 4 (1); 1973: 155–163.
19. T. Ghaye and S. Lillyman, *Reflection: Principles and Practice for Healthcare Professionals* (Salisbury: Mark Allen Publishing, 2000).
20. P. Vaill, *Learning As a Way of Being: Strategies for Survival in a World of Permanent White Water* (San Francisco, CA: Jossey-Bass, 1996).
21. T. Boydell, M. Leary, D. Megginson and M. Pedler, *Developing The Developers* (London: Association for Management Education & Development, 1991).
22. J. Edmonstone, Action learning and organisation development, in *Action Learning in Practice*, Fourth edition, ed. Mike Pedler (Farnham: Gower Publishing, 2011) 285–295.
23. W. French and C. Bell, *Organisation Development: Behavioural Science Interventions for Organisation Improvement* (Englewood Cliffs, NJ: Prentice-Hall, 1999).
24. George Weiland and Hilary Leigh (Eds.), *Changing Hospitals* (London: Tavistock Publications, 1971).
25. G. Wills and C. Oliver, Measuring the return on investment from management action learning, *Management Development Review* 9 (1); 1996: 17–21.
26. F. Furedi, *Where Have All The Intellectuals Gone? Confronting Twenty-First Century Philistinism* (London: Continuum Press, 2004).
27. V. Garrow, *OD Past Present And Future Working Paper 22 Institute for Employment Studies* (Brighton: University of Brighton, 2009).
28. J. Edmonstone and M. Havergal, The death (And Rebirth?) of OD, *Health Manpower Management* 21 (1); 1995: 28–33.
29. R. Revans, Evidence of learning; A study of manufacturing industry, in *Belgium Where Action Learning Was Tried In 1968* (Manchester: Manchester School of Management, University of Manchester Institute of Science & Technology, Occasional Paper, 1988).

2

How does action learning differ from other development approaches?

You must learn by doing the thing. For though you think you know it, you have no certainty until you try.

(Sophocles)

Action learning can be seen as part of a wider growth of interest in action-based approaches to learning and research in the management and organisational fields that contrast with more positivist approaches and focus instead on '*meaningful knowledge produced in the service of, and in the midst of, action*' (1), in contrast to more theoretical knowledge. It is marked by the powerful emphasis that it gives to the people who actually own their problems, together with a healthy scepticism towards the viewpoints and advice given by all types of expert.

There may be a potential danger, however, of confusing action learning with other seemingly similar development approaches. On occasion sometimes disparaged as simply '*learning-by-doing*', action learning is much more than this. Although it may share some characteristics with other kinds of group work, it is a unique process.

So action learning is **not**:

- ***A discussion group***: In a discussion group the rule is simply to follow the topic that is under discussion. In an action learning set the focus remains on the person and the problem or issue that they have brought to the set (2).
- ***A formal meeting***: Action learning sets do not have a role for a chair or convenor and where they do have an agenda then it is one that is created only by the set members themselves. In two senses the set may slightly mirror more formal meetings by having tight time constraints and in producing a record of the decisions made or the action points agreed, but the focus of set meetings is completely around the focal set member's issue and their need for support and challenge in addressing it.

- ***A seminar*:** In a seminar a presentation is made on the basis of well-prepared material for a discussion within a group. Seminar papers are concerned with the world '*out-there*', but action learning sets are concerned with the world '*out-there*' only insofar as it is related to the individual set member, their particular context and the specific issue which they bring to the set. There is also usually a lack of spontaneity in a seminar and the rules of discussion are seldom directed towards helping the particular person who gave the seminar paper and are still less based upon action as a result of the discussion.
- ***A simulation*:** Simulations (such as an '*organisation laboratory*'), case studies and games ultimately have no real consequences for the actions decided upon and taken, so the degree of commitment on the part of the participants is necessarily less. Moreover, there is the ever-present possibility for unnecessary rivalry and competition. These activities do involve analysis, but this is largely theoretical in nature, and participants hold no real responsibility for any decisions taken. Without any real element of risk and without the possibility of seeing the consequences of such decisions, there is little scope for true learning.
- ***Self-development group*:** An action learning set is different from a self-development group because its concern is with, and attention to, action. A set is less concerned with issues of self-discovery and much more with acting on the learning gained from reflection on experiences. The focus is therefore on making a difference '*out-there*', although '*in-here*' is inevitably involved in the process of reflection.
- ***A support group*:** The clue is in the name. The danger in such groups is that they emphasise support only, to the exclusion of challenge, and there is therefore a danger of a form of cosy collusion developing as the group comes to resemble a '*vicar's tea-party*' – a pleasant social gathering and a holiday from the rigours of organisational life. Action learning's emphasis on what set members will do when they return to the workplace avoids this.
- ***A blame group*:** Attacking others (as '*villains*') and blaming them for particular individual and organisational problems, while self-idealising (portraying ourselves as '*heroes*') is a sterile activity and unlikely to lead to any real change.
- ***Teambuilding*:** Members of an action learning set typically tend not to be members of an intact team, but rather to be individuals who are bringing a work-based issue from a unique and idiosyncratic local context, to be worked on with help from other set members. A team usually has a well-defined group task and team members work for the benefit of that task, which they have to complete, and which, of course, is the rationale for them being together. By contrast, an action learning set tends largely to work on the future actions of individual set members.
- ***Outdoor development*:** While outdoor development does provide participants with challenges and the need to improvise and to devise creative approaches to such challenges, the problems which are addressed are not real work problems – indeed they could be said to be, in Revans' terms '*puzzles*' to which there is ultimately a correct answer.
- ***A taskforce or project team*:** The points made above regarding teambuilding also apply here. Furthermore, the emphasis in an action learning set is as much on learning as it is on action. A project team's membership is completely defined by the task it undertakes and that work is driven by the intended '*deliverables*', by progress '*milestones*' and by

desired outcomes. A project team is then dissolved once the particular project is completed, while an action learning set can potentially continue for as long as the set members themselves believe that they are gaining something useful from the experience.

- ***Quality circles*:** As with task forces and project teams, quality circles are focused on a specific task and usually neither have the power to implement nor the expectation that they will then take action – they are therefore advisory, rather than executive. Learning that occurs in such groups is incidental to the primary task.
- ***Thinking environment*:** This approach involves identifying and fostering behaviours that develop independent thinking. It assumes that attentive and respectful listening encourages people to think for themselves and that blockages to such thinking are based upon personal assumptions that can be removed by incisive questioning. As such, as an approach it is supportive of coaching, mentoring, team development and also of action learning, with which it shares many underlying assumptions.
- ***Professional supervision*:** There are clear parallels between action learning and peer-group professional supervision, not least the emphasis on the need to build trust; the emphasis on confidentiality; work-focused regular meetings; the sometimes uncomfortable nature of self-review and an encouragement for individuals to develop personal solutions to their workplace problems by challenging their own practice. The major difference between action learning and other group supervision formats is the replacement of an individual professional supervisor by '*supervision*' from a group of experienced peers (4).
- ***Group therapy*:** This involves exploring personal issues at the expense of addressing work-related issues. There is no aim in an action learning set to '*peel away*' layers of personal meaning. Talking is not seen to be enough – action learning set members need to make the leap from intention to action. The intention is to learn from reflection on experience in order to undertake further action, so the focus is pragmatic and the ultimate power lies with each set member, rather than with the facilitator and other set members.
- ***Coaching, mentoring and counselling*:** Action learning is a group process, rather than a one-to-one process. A set member presenting their issue to the set can expect to be listened to and to have questions and comments aimed at helping them, but they should never expect personal counselling because this is not what is on offer in the set. While set members can discover in action learning a conducive context for exploring such personal problems and discovering underlying personal issues, they are less likely to find in the set the personal therapy which they might want in order to deal with their individual psychological problems.
- ***Communities of practice*:** A community of practice is a group of people who share a profession, occupation or interest. It can evolve naturally due to members' common interest in a domain or area or can be created specifically with the goal of gaining knowledge related to the particular field. Through the process of sharing information and experience within the group, members learn from each other and have the opportunity to develop both personally and professionally.

Although there are therefore overlaps and some similarities between action learning and communities of practice, there are also important differences, as shown below:

Communities of practice	Action learning	
Description	A principle or theory, with little explanation of methods	A methodology with less theory
Goal	Stewarding a domain	Problem-solving
Process	Analysing differences in each other's practice	Sharing experiences and focusing on necessary action
Participation	Varying levels of voluntary participation	A fixed group of people over a defined period of time
Activity	A mix of activity	Addressing problems, questioning, reflection, review and planning action
Period	Can extend over a long time	A determined period of time (3)

Nonetheless, action learning can be complementary to, and supportive of, such developmental approaches as coaching, mentoring, professional supervision, practice development and communities of practice.

- ***Action research***: Given the similarity of the names, action learning and action research can superficially be seen as being one and the same. Certainly both are grounded in tackling real organisational or societal issues. Even though action learning and action research may look broadly similar, the two have fundamentally different approaches. Action research is generally a cyclical and iterative research approach, conducted within specific and often practical organisational contexts, undertaken with rigour and understanding, so as to constantly generate new knowledge and to refine practice. It is deliberate, systematic, rigorous, scrutinised, verifiable and always made public through publication and/or oral reports. In contrast, action learning does not require that learners collect and analyse data in such a rigorous and formal manner, as is the case with action research.

  Action learning is a more general approach to learning, in which research is not the primary aim and the issue addressed may not involve any formal research at all. The individual is undertaking learning from concrete experience and from critical reflection on that experience, through small group discussion, trial and error, discovery and learning from one another. Learning is therefore a group process, yet each set member draws different learning from their different experiences. Action learning is thus focused on learning for those directly involved in a challenge or question, whereas in action research a team of people draw collective learning from a collective experience. Action research seeks to distil wider knowledge from specific issues, to be shared with a wider audience (5).

  The difference between action learning and action research is therefore the same as that between learning and research. Action research can even be seen, in a certain light, to include action learning, and indeed has been described as an unusual and non-directive form of the same, which puts the responsibility for both action and research into the hands of those directly experiencing the challenges (6). Action learning can be distinguished, ultimately, by the sovereignty that it gives to those who actually face challenges and by its scepticism regarding experts of all kinds.

So, while action learning is not any of these approaches, it does share a number of features with some of them, and especially with action research, communities of practice, thinking environment and professional supervision. These examples of '*good company*' to action learning have been characterised as follows (7):

- They are all dialectic rather than didactic or classroom-based.
- They develop contextualised and useful theory rather than test de-contextualised and impartial theory which is uncontaminated by practice.
- They invite learners to be active participants, leading often to change in the self and in the system in question.
- They emphasise reflection-in-action, rather than reflection-on-action.
- They emphasise capability over competence (see below).
- Learning tends to be facilitated rather than taught.
- They espouse the development of double-loop rather than just single-loop learning.
- They welcome the contribution of tacit knowledge to learning.
- Their learning outcomes are more often practice-based rather than academic.
- They are comfortable with tentativeness rather than certainty.

> Debate doesn't really change things. It gets you bogged down. If you can address or re-open the subject with something new, something from a different angle, then there is some hope.
>
> *(Seamus Heaney)*

REFERENCES

1. J. Raelin, Preface to a special issue "the action dimension in management": Diverse approaches to research, teaching and development, *Management Learning* 30 (2); 1999: 115–125.
2. M. Pedler and C. Abbott, *Facilitating Action Learning: A Practitioner's Guide* (Maidenhead: Open University Press, 2013).
3. J. Lave and E. Wenger, *Situated Learning: Legitimate Peripheral Participation* (Cambridge: Cambridge University Press, 1991).
4. M. Haith and K. Whittingham, How to use action learning sets to support nurses, *Nursing Times*, 108 (18/19); 2012: 12–14.
5. C. Rigg and D. Coghlan, Action learning and action research: Revisiting similarities, differences, complementarities and whether it matters, *Action Learning Research & Practice* 13 (3); 2016: 201–203.
6. P. Clark, *Action Research and Organisational Change* (London: Harper & Row, 1972).
7. J. Raelin, The action modalities: Action learning's good company, in *Action Learning in Practice*, Fourth edition, ed. Mike Pedler (Farnham: Gower Publishing, 2011) 369–379.

3

Action learning as ethos and method

Action learning is best considered as both an **ethos** (or a general way of thinking about learning and a framework with a set of values and beliefs of learner empowerment, participation and friendship at the core) and a **method** – or more accurately a variety of methods (essentially a set of experiential and action-focused practices). There is broad agreement on the main features of action learning, but there are significant variations in its practice (1).

ACTION LEARNING AS ETHOS

> What is the sense of knowing things that are useless? They will not prepare us for our unavoidable encounter with the unknown.
>
> *(Carlos Casteneda)*

Reg Revans, who developed action learning, based it upon a moral philosophy which involved:

- Honesty about ones' self
- Starting from a state of ignorance – from accepting a position of not knowing in order to find and to address fresh questions
- Action as being imperative for learning – and not just thought
- All done in a spirit of friendship
- For the overall and ultimate purpose of doing good in the world (2)

Action learning also has an epistemological base, epistemology being the theory of the origin, nature, methods and limits of knowledge. Much of that ethos has been described in Chapter 1. Building on the original work of Lyotard, Pedler et al. (1) also propose a '*cognitive map*' indicating where action learning fits. It is a framework for thinking about the positioning of action learning based upon three positions, as shown in Figure 3.1.

The positions are:

- ***Speculative:*** This is learning for its own sake, unconcerned with any application to practice and concerned largely with theoretical rigour.

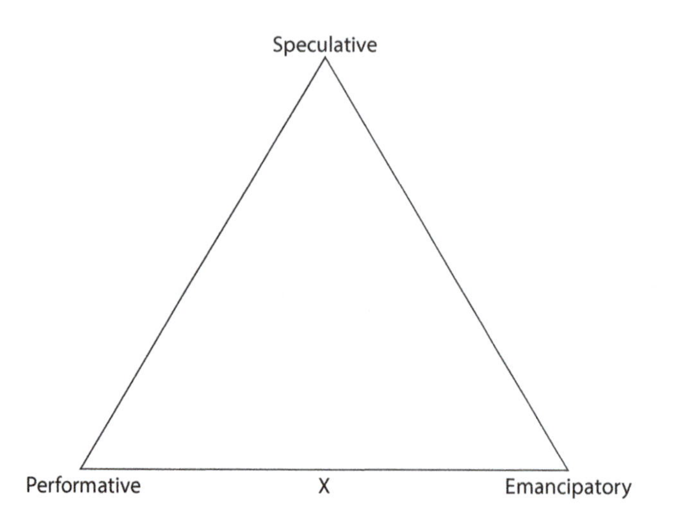

Figure 3.1 A cognitive map of action learning.

- ***Emancipatory***: This is learning that helps to overcome oppression and to attain the highest human potential. It is concerned with the holistic development of the person in the world.
- ***Performative***: This is learning that helps with action in the world; that resolves problems and produces better services and goods. It is concerned with improving, with modernising and with enhanced performance.

Revans' personal journey began as a physicist working with Lord Rutherford at the Cavendish Laboratory at Cambridge University, so he was originally located at the Speculative point of Lyotard's triangle. In the 1950s and 1960s he became concerned with practical problems in coal mines, schools, factories and hospitals as he operated in an '*operational research*' mode and so he moved to a point located between Speculative and Performative. Latterly, as he became more interested in the influence of human action and learning on the improvement of organisations and systems and so recognised the limits of purely scientific approaches to human problems, action learning became positioned at point X between Performative and Emancipatory, and this is where most action learning is currently located. Reflecting this, Pedler et al. (1) have commented that:

> Action learning is optimistic, humanistic, engaging, but also pragmatic and sceptical, suspicious of canonical ideas (and the experts who trade in them) and distrustful of speculative knowledge untested in action.

The development of Critical Action Learning (see later in this chapter) moves the focus again towards a point located between Speculative and Emancipatory, although the potential danger of this location is that greater analytical power may be achieved, but at the expense of an emphasis on both action and reality testing.

Pedler at al also refer to two '*moral syndromes*' (3) of the ***Guardians*** (or '*keepers of the sacred flame*' who anathematise deviations from the original ideas of action learning's originator, Reg Revans) and the ***Traders*** (connecting-up different aspects of action learning practice, exploring variations, learning from both and modifying their own practice).

The challenge, they claim, is to be both Guardians (of the action learning ethos) and Traders (of the different methods).

Recent commentators have also seen the increasing necessity of developing the ability of learning how to learn for economic, social and political reasons. It has been suggested that, using the notion of '*figure and ground*' derived from Gestalt psychology, achieving immediate learning goals is the '*figure*' of any learning activity, but the '*ground*' is the development of intuitive understanding of, and expertise at, the learning process itself (4). In other words, in the Interpretive and Associative learning modes mentioned in Chapter 1. As we learn what to do, we also change how we know, and how we come to know.

> That is what learning is. You suddenly understand something you've understood all your life, but in a new way.
>
> *(Doris Lessing)*

The other key aspects of the ethos of action learning are:

$$L > C$$

Professor Reg. Revans, the originator of action learning, began his career as a scientist and had a liking for expressing core ideas in formulae. One such was $L > C$, where L is the rate of individual and organisational learning and C is the rate of individual and organisational change. The formula, which is an almost Darwinian law of organisational and personal survival, implies that both individuals and organisations need to learn at least as fast as, but ideally faster than, the speed at which things change around them, if they are to have any hope of keeping up. Organisations and people that embody and express only past ideas are not learning and unless they adapt through learning then they will become extinct. Education and training programmes that teach people to be proficient in yesterday's techniques and methods simply do not equip people for meeting today and tomorrow's challenges and opportunities, but rather make them '*walk backwards into the future*'.

> You always got to be prepared, but you never know for what.
>
> *(Bob Dylan, 'Sugar Babe')*

$$L = P + Q$$

Sometimes known as the Learning Equation, here L stands for Learning, P equals Programmed knowledge and Q is Questioning insight. Learning is therefore seen to be made up of two main elements and the first, ***Programmed knowledge***, is seen as comprising of two aspects – external and internal. ***External programmed knowledge*** is pre-packaged and recorded information and knowledge prepared for learners by experts, and is contained in a range of '*products*' such as textbooks, manuals, checklists, algorithms, lecture notes, online material, and so on. These have all been produced in order to capture what has already been learned, as a means of avoiding the learner reinventing the wheel. ***Internal programmed knowledge*** is made up of an individual's personal mind-set or mental models derived from their prior experience. ***Questioning insight*** is the process of active listening, questioning and reflecting, leading to review and revision of personal experience at the edge of understanding.

Questioning Insight arises from inquiry and from powerful questions about personal experience. It is most useful where there is a limited degree of understanding around a problem, or where the problem area is rapidly changing. It is '*frontier learning*' – taking place at the edge of understanding. It does not cumulatively build knowledge, but rather helps to reorganise understanding and to see it anew. Participants in action learning largely learn from generating insights, rather than simply collecting knowledge and advice, although this also occurs.

There are real tensions between P and Q. P, for example, starts and finishes with answers and with instructions, while Q explores what P cannot achieve and forces it to change. If P is pushed it ultimately produces answers that are harmonious and technically complete. Q creates more questions than answers, and ultimately finishes with a new question. A Q '*state of mind*' recognises the value of P and accepts it as a co-partner in learning. P, however, only recognises other forms of P.

Nonetheless, there are dangers in setting-up P and Q as diametrically opposed states, for they are both necessary for effective learning. Providing learners with P that is irrelevant to the particular issue that they face can be disastrous, but so can unfocused Q – as a form of navel contemplation. Both P and Q are required because neither can be useful in and of themselves. Revans maintained that action learning did not reject all formal instruction, but that '*it merely recognises that, however necessary such instruction may be, it is by no means sufficient*' (5).

One useful way of seeing the relationship between P and Q is shown in Figure 3.2.

In this figure a problem or issue (Q.1) is explored and it becomes obvious that some Programmed Knowledge (external or internal) is relevant to addressing this problem. After applying this (P.1) the original problem is reformulated (Q.2). In turn, further Programmed Knowledge (P.2) is applied, leading to further clarification of the problem (Q.3) and so on. When you begin with Questioning Insight, you often find that some of the existing Programmed

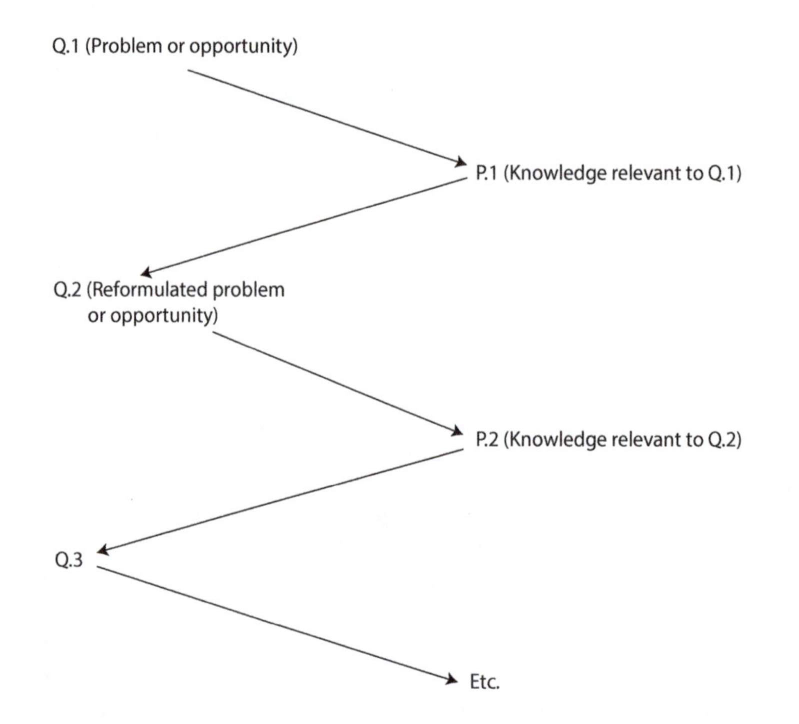

Figure 3.2 Relationship between P and Q.

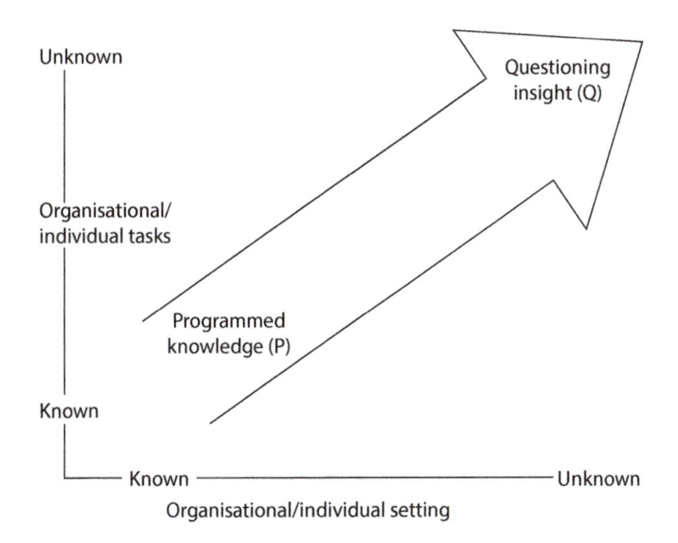

Figure 3.3 Programmed knowledge, questioning insight and the part of change.

Knowledge seemingly related to the problem being addressed is of little value, and that there therefore may be new Programmed Knowledge that must be acquired or developed. The problem situation often does need the application of relevant Programmed Knowledge – but only on a '*just-in-time*' basis. The dangerous alternative is that sets can '*close in*' on themselves and not seek the other perspectives which relevant P might bring.

Getting the balance right between Programmed Knowledge and Questioning Insight is a major challenge. Too much P and not enough Q can lead to a top-down and didactic delivery of knowledge – therefore repeating the problems with traditional learning identified in Chapter 1. An over-concentration on Q at the expense of P means that people may end up '*reflecting on their reflections*' and pooling their ignorance without any access to knowledge relevant to their particular problem situation. The faster the rate of change that people and organisations experience (see L $>$ C), the more quickly P then become out-of-date, and therefore the more important Q becomes as a means of producing new understanding of the changed situation. This is shown in Figure 3.3.

Figure 3.3. suggests that in those situations where the tasks or challenges that an individual or organisation has to undertake are well-known, and where the setting in which those tasks take place is familiar, then P will largely suffice. However, where the setting and tasks facing both organisations and individuals are both largely unknown, then there is a corresponding greater need for Q. This is the state of affairs facing most individuals and most organisations in the twenty-first century.

Balancing learning and task cycles

In most work organisations (and most probably in life generally) there is what has been called an '*action-fixated non-learning cycle*' (6) in operation for most people for most of the time. As Figure 3.4. shows, people observe a particular situation and in a '*rush to judgement*' almost immediately devise an explanation or theory in order to explain what is happening, which then forms the basis of the action which they take in order to deal with the situation.

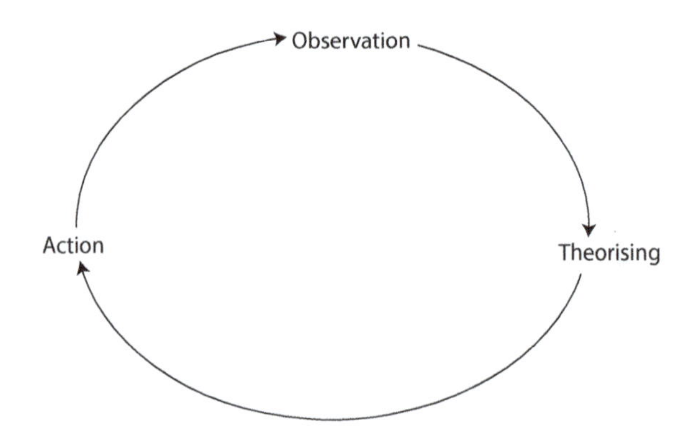

Figure 3.4 Action-fixated non-learning cycle.

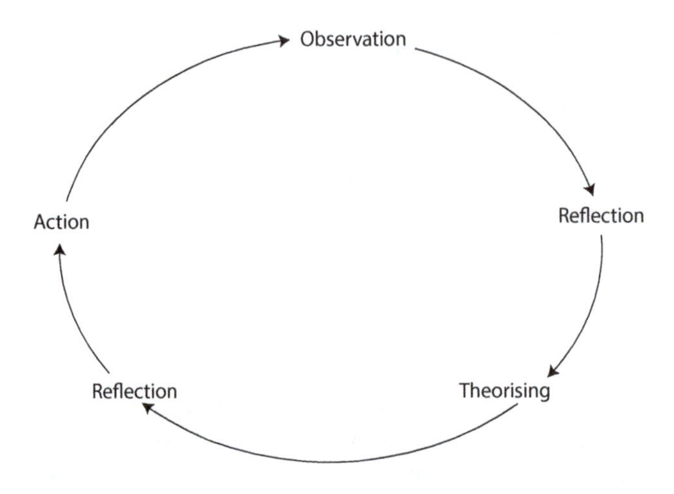

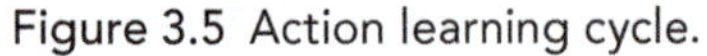
Figure 3.5 Action learning cycle.

However, taking action and believing that you have learned from it are not the same as taking action and then reviewing that experience in depth, with the help of colleagues and really learning from it. A second activity cycle – of learning – is necessary, and is shown in Figure 3.5.

This activity cycle emphasises the importance of reviewing past and current experience and concluding what has been learned from it, as the basis for planning what comes next. The reviewing, concluding and thinking about results components of the two cycles are often either forgotten or are short-circuited in a culture of '*busy-ness*' and in order to get things done quickly. However, attention to this part of the process is the key to more effective problem-solving and to successful individual learning and development, and is the reason that action learning insists on the need for reflection and review. Balancing the tensions between learning and delivering tangible results is therefore a challenge in action learning.

Single- and double-loop learning

Single-loop learning is both adaptive and tactical – simply solving an immediate problem – and thus represents incremental change (7–9). It asks '*Are we doing things right?*' and occurs when goals, values, frameworks and strategies are taken for granted and so rarely change.

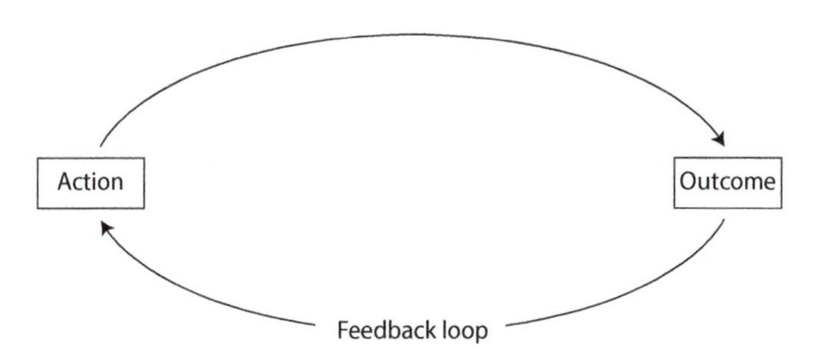

Figure 3.6 Single-loop learning.

It improves the status quo by narrowing the gap between desired and actual positions. It is effectively error detection and correction and the maintenance of a steady state, operating like a thermostat on a boiler. If it gets too hot, the thermostat tells the boiler to cool it and the boiler changes its actions to produce a different outcome. People similarly receive such feedback and so change their actions, but not always their minds, as shown in Figure 3.6. It is the world of everyday, normal, natural '*in-the-box*' thinking. Such learning tends to leave organisational objectives and processes largely unchallenged and therefore unchanged.

Double-loop learning is where minds are changed as a result of the feedback received. It asks '*Are we doing the right things?*' and so it calls into question the very nature of the course already plotted and the feedback loops that are used to maintain that course. For example, we may conclude that a continuing failure to get the outcomes we desire means that we might need to look at our deeper and more fundamental assumptions and conditions regarding the situation in which we find ourself. When a colleague repeatedly rejects our requests for help, or when repeated attempts to answer a question fail, then we may decide that a deeper enquiry is therefore necessary, in which we reframe thinking beyond the '*more of*' and '*less of*' approaches. We may need to consider, for example, whether we really understand the problem situation or in what light we may be seen by that colleague. These deeper questions which challenge fundamental assumptions with regard to goals and strategies are typical of action learning and prompt more fundamental change within an individual and a system. Double-loop learning (as shown in Figure 3.7) is less normal and less comfortable as it challenges assumptions, questions taken for granted and decisions and potentially stimulates conflict. It represents '*out-of-the-box*' thinking. Potentially, it can lead to a redefining of an organisation's

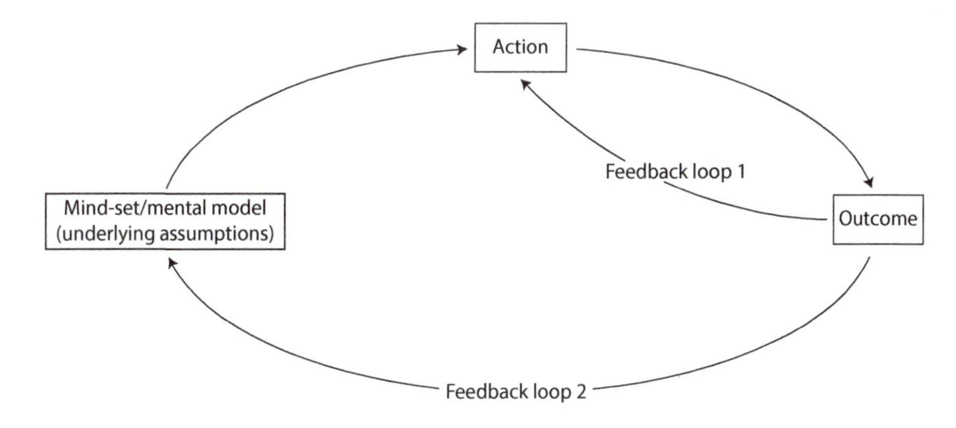

Figure 3.7 Double-loop learning.

goals, norms, policies, procedures and structures, and is therefore both strategic and generative. It would apply, for example, to a fundamental service redesign and reconfiguration.

Here are examples of single and double-loop learning based on the obstetrics clinical specialty in a hospital. With ***single-loop learning*** the hospital examines its care of obstetrics patients and, through a clinical audit, it finds a number of gaps between the established standards, which are derived from evidence-based guidelines, and the actual practice. A series of meetings are held in order to discuss the guidelines; changes are then made to working procedures and reporting and feedback on practice are enhanced. The changes increase the number of patients who are receiving appropriate and timely care.

In the case of ***double-loop learning***, while reviewing obstetric care, some patients are interviewed in depth. From this, it emerges that the issues that concern women are largely to do with such factors as convenience of access, the quality of information provided to them, continuity of care and the interpersonal aspects of the patient-professional relationship. As a result of this, obstetric care is radically reconfigured to a system of midwife-led teams in order to give priority to these matters. The standards derived from the evidence-based guidelines are not ignored, but instead are included in a reframed version of values and interactions.

The ladder of inference

Inferring is largely an automatic and unconscious process (10,11). People have to operate most of the time using higher-level abstraction in order to process the huge amount of information which they gather through their senses. Thus, assumptions and attributions about others are actually extrapolations from perceived data at various levels of abstraction – a ladder of inference, where the higher the rung on the ladder, the more abstract and less reliable is the inference (Figure 3.8).

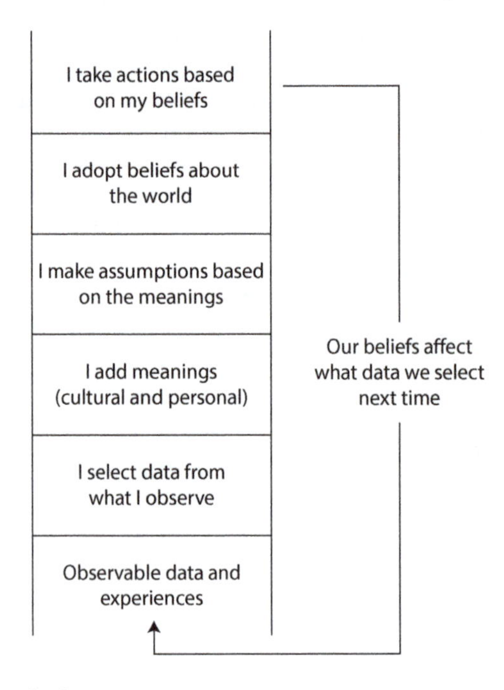

Figure 3.8 The ladder of inference.

In the course of a human lifetime our mind-sets of attitudes and beliefs become reinforced by our selective attention to events. Attention is most often paid to confirming, rather than disconfirming data. Most of the time this is a natural and helpful process, as it helps individuals to avoid information overload and the continuous reappraisal of both people and situations. However, it also means that we operate for much of the time on the basis of our biases and prejudices. Thus no two people usually experience the same event in the same way and so our natural mental '*short-cuts*' – our assumptions, expectations and biases – can prove to be unhelpful at times. As Simon and Garfunkel sang '*A man sees what he wants to see and disregards the rest.*'

Such mind-sets could include, for example:

There is somewhere a single right answer, if only I could find it.
It's important to be rational and logical at all times. Imagination is "soft and fluffy" and I'm not that kind of person.
It's important to discover what the rules are and to play by them.
I need to have an agreed plan before I can go any further.
That sounds fuzzy and ambiguous – I don't go there.
That doesn't fall within my remit, so I don't go there.

Problems frequently arise from not testing our attributions about other people's behaviour. The higher the level of inference, the more difficult it is to be explicit about our thinking processes, and, in threatening situations, it often becomes much more difficult. Very often, when things go wrong, we attribute to others our own weaknesses, assuming that we all fail for the same reasons. We seek to protect ourselves, and the others involved, by not telling them the negative attributions that we are making about them and this is typically considered to be the '*right*' thing to do. Unfortunately, by avoiding confrontation and leaving such attributions untested, they can become self-fulfilling prophecies, even if inaccurate. For example, if I assume someone is autocratic and behave to protect myself from her '*autocratic*' decisions, such as avoiding discussion of important issues with her, then she is likely to end up acting autocratically because of what she sees as my untrustworthy behaviour!

So, from our experience, we select certain data to which we add meanings based on our prior personal and cultural experience and these form the basis of the assumptions that we then make and the conclusions which we draw. These conclusions enable us to adopt beliefs about the world upon which we base our actions. This is a '*self-sealing*' process, as the beliefs we adopt then powerfully affect the data selected next time. Only by breaking the reinforcement, examining and challenging the assumptions, can deeper double-loop learning take place – and action learning provides a means by which this can happen.

Unlearning

The centrality and importance of learning is a constant within Western societies and indeed action learning might be seen as a manifestation of that state. Such a viewpoint can be seen to be embodied in the '*banking*' model of learning as something that simply gradually accumulates over time (12). Yet, in fact, action learning challenges this by a strong consideration of the need for unlearning. The dialogue which takes place between set members offers a means of interrupting and breaching well-established patterns of thinking and behaviour, as redundant mind-sets are re-evaluated, re-positioned and embodied within a wider repertoire of possible responses.

This is not simply about forgetting, but paradoxically is concerned with advancing by slowing-down, by stepping-back and by letting-go from prior understanding that may limit the future. As set members become more aware of what they do, this potentially disruptive process can, of course, be experienced as discomforting, as individuals see the ways in which they may sabotage themselves, but also liberating.

It has been suggested that unlearning is particularly apposite for addressing wicked problems, many of which are located in health, social and community care (13) and that a Critical Action Learning orientation (see below) may, by admitting the importance of '*not-knowing*' and '*non-action*' (effectively an emphasis on rumination and incubation) create a space for completely new questions and possibilities to emerge. '*Sleeping on it*' can foster this process of incubation and allow the unconscious mind to get to work (14).

The Principle Of Insufficient Mandate: Revans maintained that:

> Those unable to change themselves cannot change what goes on around them. (5)

This simple proposition has profound implications as it means that the starting-point for change lies with each individual and that all such individuals, regardless of experience or status, are responsible for their own self-development. It also implies that the development of such individuals is the real precondition for the development of organisations. Finally, it also means that, in periods of rapid and complex change, a person's previous experience, no matter how comprehensive and extensive, is likely to be of very limited relevance.

ACTION LEARNING AS METHOD

> The unexamined life is not worth living.
>
> *(Socrates)*

Action learning is definitely not a '*recipe-book*' approach but is flexible enough to be adapted to a huge variety of different settings and challenges. Common to all the variants on the action learning theme is a set of '*components*'. These are:

Work: The ongoing role or job of a set member, with all the real-time issues, opportunities and experiences which the workplace setting offers.

Action: The centrepiece of action learning is action. There is no learning without action and no action without learning. The action to be taken serves as the '*engine*' that drives the learning process, promoting critical reflection and learning.

An individual set member: Each individual has particular life and work experiences, preferences and styles and faces workplace and personal challenges. They voluntarily opt to be part of a peer group of people addressing similar challenges. Each set member brings with them their own particular ***context*** (or unique work setting), ***characteristics*** (their personal styles and attributes) and ***challenge*** (their workplace problem, challenge or question).

Problem: The particular real-time '*presenting*' (15) or '*starting*' issue, challenge or question that the set member has previously agreed with their sponsor in their work organisation and that the set member wants to work on in both set meetings and back in the workplace. The problem will not only be salient to the set member but also to their organisation and hopefully also to other set members. The problem may deal with strategic issues (i.e. what to do) or operational/tactical issues (i.e. how to do it) and may well evolve and change as the work of the set progresses. It may not always be easily recognisable or explainable and often can appear '*messy*', especially at the outset – that is, not simply neat and easily solvable. Often it is marked by some sense of a repeating pattern. The intention is always to achieve tangible progress within the time available as part of the action learning programme. Some sets may work on different aspects of a single shared and common problem, while others may work on a variety of different issues.

Information: Knowledge acquired by set members and generated by individual search and research and from interaction amongst set members. It involves facts and data in relation to the problem or question derived from policy, research, reports, models, books, journal articles, workshops and so on – together with that information which is generated from set members listening carefully to each other.

The action learning set: The small and stable group of between four and seven or eight colleagues, voluntarily formed together and committed to a supportive but challenging partnership, meeting over a fixed or agreed timescale in order to help action to be taken on challenges to which there are no readily available answers. The set is committed to learning from the exploration of such challenges. It is a collective space for thinking and working where every set member acts as a consultant, advisor and devil's advocate to every other set member in a supportive partnership. There is no assigned leader within the set. Every set is unique because of the individual differences between the set members, their wider contexts and the specific challenges which they face.

Sponsor: An influential senior manager or professional who also has ownership of the set member's issue; who desires progress to be made and who has agreed with the set member that there are benefits to them from being involved in action learning. Occasionally the term '*client*' is used instead of sponsor. Sometimes sponsors are the set member's line manager, but there is also real value in the sponsor being an '*off-line*' senior person who is willing to act as a mentor and to give time to the personal and professional development of the set member. This sponsor will have discussed and agreed on the issue with the individual set member; will give priority to the set member's regular attendance at set meetings and will provide ongoing support and challenge at work, which might include, for example '*opening doors*' to other departments/functions/ professions/organisations. This sponsor role might also involve, for example, attendance at start-up, mid-point and end-point events in a programme, and will clearly involve some time-commitment on the sponsor's part. The sponsor provides the set member with clarity, support, guidance, and advice. They are an early port of call for reporting-back on set member's findings and in helping with the evaluation process.

Champion: Within the wider organisational system there is also a role for a champion or champions of the action learning approach. Typically, this is an individual or a group of people who have benefitted from previous set membership. Such a senior individual or group act as an advocate for the action learning process, operate as a broker, linking set members to key people and also ensure ongoing momentum.

Facilitator: Each set will have a facilitator – a person who sets the scene and acts as an initiator, role model and catalyst for the set meetings and who is particularly active in the early days of the set. Their primary responsibility is to support the process of learning, including demonstrating exemplary listening and questioning skills, ensuring that everyone is engaged and managing time within the set meetings. As the set matures the facilitator may take a more '*occasional*' role. Some sets may eventually become self-facilitating or may be so from the outset, with facilitation shared between set members.

Process: This involves observation of the problem situation or issue; reflection; the forming of explanations or theories and the taking of action. Factual information about the issue is gathered on an ongoing basis. Reflection and theorising take place before, during and after set meetings and action takes place back in the workplace.

Time-frame: Problems are considered with a defined period of time and this necessarily gives rise to action learning programmes having a beginning, middle and end.

> The more we cling to past practices, the more we deepen the crisis and prevent solutions.
>
> *(Margaret Wheatley)*

VARIANTS OF ACTION LEARNING

There is no single universally agreed definition of action learning and no single '*best*' way of doing it. For example, in the United States action learning is much more structured in approach than in the UK or in Europe. Rather, it can be perceived as a family of approaches. While there is agreement on the major features of the idea, there are many variations in its practice. As a result, one of the strengths of action learning is that it is continually re-invented or re-interpreted to meet current conditions and challenges. Therefore, the definition offered in the Introduction is indeed both personal and tentative. The different variants of action learning include:

- ***'Mainstream' action learning***: This is the approach largely featured in this book and is the one most used in health, social and community care (16–18). Among the ways in which it is used are:
  - As a planned and timetabled activity which is interwoven with other aspects of a development programme, with the action learning set either ceasing at the end of the programme or being allowed or encouraged to continue, typically in a self-managed way, for as long as the set members continue to derive benefit from it.
  - As an activity introduced towards the end of a more formal and structured development programme, with the anticipation that the programme participants would form sets as a way of continuing their development and so bridge the '*learning transfer*' gap between the programme and work.
  - As a discrete development activity in its own right, often in a particular professional field, geographical patch or with a focus on an emerging issue or new role, and neither relying upon nor continuing the momentum of a formal programme (19).
- ***Business-driven action learning***: This is similar to mainstream action learning, the major difference being that the issues which the set members work on are not chosen by them but are organisationally-derived and reflect the organisation's current and future strategic and operational priorities (20,21). This approach emphasises the integration of a business and results-focused orientation with individual development and team effectiveness as the

set members pursue measurable results. It therefore requires major support from senior leaders and managers to set up and to sustain. In an ideal world the set members would probably be choosing such issues anyway, provided that they were familiar with them. While this variant is undoubtedly superficially attractive to organisations, there are also the risks that:

- What is seen by the organisation as a '*presenting*' issue may have its roots in a more challenging area, where the organisation may not necessarily wish to go.
- The set member may, as a result of participation in the set, come up with an '*unacceptable finding*', i.e. a conclusion which is at odds with conventional wisdom within the organisation; that challenges established interests or that involves the deployment of resources that are unobtainable.
- Moreover, this approach also runs the potential risk of action learning being regarded simply as a tool or means towards an end.

- ***Virtual action learning***: Faced with the busy life which most professionals and managers lead, the question has been raised as to whether virtual action learning sets can offer a valid alternative to the face-to-face interaction which most sets provide (22–24). Virtual action learning is therefore an emerging and fairly new form (beginning in the late 1990s) conducted in a virtual environment using collaborative communication technology, rather than by set members meeting face-to-face.

  Six potential forms of virtual action learning are shown below:

	Synchronous	Asynchronous
	(Participants interact in same finite time period	(Participants interact at different time periods)
Text	Instant messaging	Email/text messaging On-line discussion
Audio	Live telephone/audio conferencing	Audio recordings
Audio-visual	Skype – web-based conferencing	Video recordings

The ***advantages*** of virtual action learning are:

- Sets can cover a wide geographical area and even be international in nature, allowing for greater diversity in set membership.
- Significant savings can be achievable in both travel time and costs.
- The non-physical presence and sense of anonymity compared with face-to-face action learning can potentially foster more openness; help to establish personal identities and speed-up the development of trust and good working relationships.
- Listening seems intensified and it becomes easier to concentrate on what is being said without the need to constantly maintain eye contact, as would be the case in a face-to-face set.
- Responses are therefore more thoughtful than in faster face-to-face dialogue.
- Voice is more '*visible*' in intonation, tone, inflection, speed and silences.

The ***disadvantages*** of virtual action learning are:

- The non-physical presence and anonymity presents a difficulty for some set members.
- The complexity of the technology – it is often not familiar or easy to use and therefore may get in the way.

- This approach is heavily dependent on the skills of the facilitator. These skills are at two levels:
  - ***Macro-level***: Creating the initial conditions necessary to set-up virtual action learning. This involves the time and effort required in selecting, training and preparing the facilitator and set members with the technology and setting-up the virtual meetings.
  - ***Micro-level***: The resources, skills and processes necessary to run virtual action learning sessions – managing both the process and the technology.

Of great importance with virtual action learning is '*netiquette*' – specific rules of behaviour which amplify the value of the approach. These include such matters as:

- For the conversation, the need to find a quiet room where the set member will not be distracted.
- Aiming for only one person to speak at a time.
- Yet, accepting interruptions because there is a need to develop trust and spontaneity.
- Seeking to apportion equal time to each individual in both issue discussion and in explorations of the issue.
- If someone seems silent during a call, aiming to bring them in.
- When an individual is reviewing the possible actions they are considering, noting down any suggestions.
- The facilitator tries to keep to the times agreed and provides notes of the session afterwards.

At present virtual action learning still remains largely experimental, pioneering and highly diverse in its many manifestations which operate in a diverse range of organisational contexts and in pursuit of a wide range of objectives. Although it seems to work well in certain contexts and offers potential for further research and use, it also raises a number of questions, such as how virtual action learning can best be facilitated and the nature of virtual group dynamics. It need not, of course, necessarily be exclusive of mainstream action learning – there could, for example, be advantages of commencing an action learning set face-to-face and then continuing it on a virtual basis.

- ***Blended action learning***: This takes place where action learning is used alongside a range of other approaches as part of a formal qualification-based programme, usually at Masters degree level (25–27). It would sit with other approaches such as lecture-based modules, an online virtual learning platform, case studies, and so on – the point being that action learning is '*blended*' with these approaches as a means of contributing towards the overall programme outcomes.
- ***Critical action learning***: This is a fairly recent approach which seeks to reveal how power relations are a significant part of action learning and of organisational life more generally (28–30). The emphasis is therefore not only on the empowerment of the individual set member, but also on the ways in which learning and action are supported, but also avoided and prevented, both within sets themselves and in work organisations, through relations of power. It assumes that power relations are an inevitable and integral part of action learning and may be represented by such examples as individual set members' risk-averse behaviour within sets; by collective defensiveness and denial and by set members' unconscious compliance with certain taken-for-grated organisational habits, norms and expectations. For example, Vince notes that while what may be desired in action learning sets is '*learning-in-action*' what may be actually evidenced is '*learning inaction*' (30).

The distinguishing features of critical action learning are:

- An emphasis on the ways that learning is supported, avoided, and/or prevented through power relations.
- The linking of questioning insight to complex emotions and to unconscious processes and relations.
- An emphasis on collective, as well as individual, reflection – that is, on organisational, political and emotional dynamics.
- Reflection which is critical of taken-for-granted assumptions with regard to the social and political forces which provide the context for work and organisations.
- A more active facilitation role than for mainstream action learning.

Critical action learning is therefore very challenging of existing power relations within organisations and can therefore be an uncomfortable experience for both set members, their organisational sponsors and the organisation itself. It is advanced as a means of correcting an unquestioning tradition, particularly in management learning, where, because leaders and managers tend to become accultured by a form of '*cultural doping*' (31) and so to share a dominant ideology and values, they are then unwilling, unlikely and seemingly unable to question such a perspective. Action learning therefore runs the risk of capture by powerful corporate interests for use as a tool – a means of effecting incremental improvements in organisational performance while still maintaining a status quo of dominance and control (32,33).

Power is everywhere; not because it embraces everything, but because it comes from everywhere.

(Michel Foucault)

- ***Self-managed action learning***: Although current good practice typically involves the use of a facilitator working with the action learning set, one variant seeks to dispense with this role (34–36). Here the term '*facilitator*' is often replaced with that of '*set manager*' and is undertaken by set members themselves. Set meetings are much more structured and less free-form than with mainstream action learning. Specifically, there are two rounds of time-slots – one is ***retrospective*** and focuses on reflection and looking back to learn the lessons of experience, while the other is ***prospective***, looking forward to identify the actions needed to move set members forward. It is less common to find self-facilitated sets, however, and there are a number of reasons for this:
  - The expectations of the set members themselves, or of their sponsors, that a facilitator role is necessary.
  - A lack of understanding among set members at the initial stage about what the process of action learning entails.
  - The need for help to enable set members to get to know and develop trust in each other at an early stage.
  - The lack of skills among the set members to self-facilitate.
  - The need for someone who holds responsibility for helping the learning process for the set.

  Self-managed sets are sometimes a viable option, particularly where the set membership is experienced and mature, perhaps drawn from membership of previous sets, so that they can work in a self-managed way. However, to do so demands:
  - A high personal commitment from all set members to attend the set meetings and to share the work of facilitation, as mutually agreed.

- Clear agreement among set members about the format to be followed for set meetings and clarity over the roles adopted.
- A high degree of honesty in reviewing each set meeting to avoid collusion or to ignore or avoid discussing possibly unhelpful behaviour.

Revans saw only a limited role for facilitators at the start-up stage of action learning – and certainly not on an ongoing basis. Even where a facilitator is in place the aim must be to make the role as redundant as possible as the set members become more mature and experienced in working together. Ultimately, the services of a facilitator are dispensable, but it is for the set to decide exactly when. Abandoning a set too early or outstaying the welcome are both dangers.

- ***Auto-action learning***: The membership of an individual in an action learning set can be supplemented by '*auto-action learning*'. Based around the questions posed in the Action Learning Problem Brief (see Part 3 of this book) the use of a mentor outside of the set provides an opportunity for reflection, learning and the devising of planned actions. This seems to speed-up learning and act as a motivator to apply experience from elsewhere to the problem situation. It also serves to build the principle of the empowerment of the problem-holder through the use of the format (the Action Learning Problem Brief) already established in use within the set. Auto-action learning involves a series of parallel relationships (set membership and mentoring) which serve to reinforce each other. The use of the structured format focuses attention both retrospectively (on learning achieved) and prospectively (on forward action). The use of such systematic headings seems to help keep a focus on motivation, learning and review (37,38).

Action learning thus appears in different organisations and in numerous different forms, much as a car is available in many different makes and styles, while still being recognisable as a car.

> I hear and I forget; I see and I remember; I do and I understand.
>
> *(Confucius)*

REFERENCES

1. M. Pedler, J. Burgoyne and C. Brook, What has action learning learned to become?, *Action Learning: Research & Practice* 2 (1); 2005: 49–68.
2. M. Pedler, Reginald Revans, in *Palgrave Change Thinkers Handbook*, eds. W. Pasmore, D. Szabla and M. Barnes (Basingstoke: Palgrave Macmillan, 2017).
3. J. Jacobs, *Systems of Survival* (New York, NY: Random House, 1992).
4. G. Claxton, Education for the learning age: A socio-cultural approach to learning to learn, in *Learning for Life in The Twenty-First Century*, eds. G. Wells and G. Claxton (Oxford: Blackwell, 2002).
5. R. Revans, *ABC of Action Learning* (Farnham: Gower Publishing, 2011).
6. B. Garratt, *The Learning Organisation* (London: Fontana-Collins, 1987).
7. C. Argyris, *Increasing Leadership Effectiveness* (New York, NY: Wiley, 1976).
8. G. Bateson, *Steps to an Ecology of Mind* (Chicago, IL: University of Chicago Press, 1972).
9. D. Schon, *The Reflective Practitioner: How Professionals Think in Action* (London: Temple Smith, 1983).

10. P. Senge, C. Roberts, B. Smith, A. Kleiner and R. Ross, *The Fifth Discipline Fieldbook: Strategies and Tools for Building a Learning Organisation* (New York, NY: Doubleday, 1994).
11. C. Argyris, *Strategy Change and Defensive Routines* (Boston, MA: Pitman Publishing, 1985).
12. J. Edmonstone, Escaping the healthcare leadership Cul-De-Sac, *Leadership in Health Services* 30 (1); 2017: 76–91.
13. C.I Brook, M. Pedler, C. Abbott and J. Burgoyne, On stopping doing those things that are not getting us to where we want to be: Unlearning and critical action learning, *Human Relations* 69 (2); 2016: 369–389.
14. G. Gregory, Developing intuition through management education, in *The Intuitive Practitioner: On the Value of not Always Knowing What One is Doing*, eds. Terry Atkinson and Guy Claxton (Buckingham: Open University Press, 2000).
15. P. Block, *Flawless Consulting: A Guide to Getting Your Expertise Used* (San Francisco, CA: Pfeiffer, 1981).
16. M. Pedler and C. Abbott, *Facilitating Action Learning: A Practitioner's Guide* (Maidenhead: McGraw-Hill/Open University Press, 2013).
17. C. Abbott and P. Taylor, *Action Learning in Social Work* (London: Sage, 2013).
18. J. Edmonstone, *Action Learning in Healthcare: A Practical Handbook* (London: Radcliffe Publishing, 2011).
19. A. Scowcroft, The problem with dissecting a frog (is that when you are finished it doesn't really look like a frog anymore), in *Clinical Leadership: A Book of Readings*, ed. John Edmonstone (Chichester: Kingsham Press, 2005), 271–291.
20. Y. Boshyk, Business-driven action learning today, in *Action Learning in Practice*, Fourth edition, ed. Mike Pedler (Farnham: Gower Publishing, 2011), 141–152.
21. Y. Boshyk (Ed.), *Business-Driven Action Learning: Global Best Practices* (London and New York: Macmillan Business & St. Martins, 2000).
22. K. Currie, J. Biggam, J. Palmer, J. and I. Corcoran, Participants' engagement with and reaction to the use of on-line action learning sets to support advanced nursing role development, *Nurse Education in Practice* 32 (3); 2012: 267–272.
23. M. Dickenson, M. Pedler and J. Burgoyne, Virtual action learning: Practices and challenges, *Action Learning: Research & Practice* 7 (1); 2010: 59–72.
24. M. Goodman and J.-A. Stewart, Virtual action learning, in *Action Learning in Practice*, Fourth edition, ed. Mike Pedler (Farnham: Gower Publishing, 2011), 153–161.
25. G. Boak, Blending P and Q: Incorporating action learning in a master's programme, *Action Learning: Research & Practice* 8 (2); 2011: 165–172.
26. J. Edmonstone and J. Robson, Blending-in: The contribution of action learning to a masters programme in human resources in health, *International Journal of Human Resource Development and Management* 13 (1); 2013: 61–75.
27. K. Thornton and P. Yoong, The role of the blended action learning facilitator: An enabler of learning and a trusted inquisitor, *Action Learning: Research & Practice* 8 (2); 2011: 129–146.
28. K. Trehan, Critical action learning, in *Action Learning in Practice*, Fourth edition, ed. Mike Pedler (Farnham: Gower Publishing, 2011), 163–171.
29. R. Vince, Action learning and organisational learning: Power, politics and emotions in organisations, *Action Learning: Research & Practice* 1 (1); 2004: 63–78.
30. R. Vince, Learning-in-action and learning inaction: Advancing the theory and practice of critical action learning, *Action Learning: Research & Practice* 5 (2); 2008: 93–104.

31. J. Raelin, Emancipatory discourse and liberation, *Management Learning* 39 (5); 2008: 519–540.
32. H. Willmott, Management education: Provocations to a debate, *Management Learning* 25 (1); 1994: 105–106.
33. H. Willmott, Critical management learning, in *Management Learning*, eds. John Burgoyne and Mike Reynolds (London: Sage, 1997), 161–176.
34. T. Bourner, Self-managed action learning, in *Action Learning in Practice*, Fourth edition, ed. Mike Pedler (Farnham: Gower Publishing, 2011), 113–123.
35. S. O'Hara, T. Bourner and T. Webber, The practice of self-managed action learning, *Action Learning: Research & Practice* 1 (1); 2004: 29–42.
36. S. Shurville and A. Rospigliosi, Implementing blended self-managed action learning for digital entrepreneurs in higher education, *Action Learning: Research & Practice* 6 (1); 2009: 53–61.
37. A. Learmonth and M. Pedler, Auto-action learning: A tool for policy change: Building capacity across the developing regional system to improve health in the North East of England, *Health Policy* 68 (2); 2004: 169–181.
38. A. Learmonth, Action learning as a tool for developing networks and building evidence-based practice in public health, *Action Learning: Research & Practice* 2 (1); 2005: 97–104.

4

The benefits of action learning

At the level of the ***individual***, action learning provides real opportunities for personal growth and learning. Set members face real issues and challenges which they own and are committed to making real progress on them. They therefore need to reflect on how their actions, their personal style, their motivations and their values all make an impact on others. The action learning set's focus on action and review helps individuals to experiment and to try out different approaches, thereby enhancing their self-awareness. Specifically, therefore, the claims for the benefits of action learning at the individual level include:

- A greater breadth of understanding, as a basis for building relationships across an organisation or organisations and hence taking action; personal horizons are broadened through the sharing of similar situations viewed from different perspectives
- A safe environment that enables people to think about difficult situations in which they find themselves and an improved focus on what really makes a difference in such situations
- An antidote to isolation for highly specialised professionals and managers
- An opportunity to listen and to be listened to, and hence to improve personal listening skills
- An opportunity to express feelings as well as facts about the work situation
- An improved ability to make sense of ambiguous information and situations and to address complex challenges
- A chance to examine personal and organisational assumptions and to try out alternatives that free-up thinking and help to produce concrete and practical ways forward
- An enhanced capacity to understand and to initiate organisational changes and an increased readiness to take responsibility and initiative
- Individuals who are more action-focused and proactive in delivering results
- Individuals who are more reflective than emotional in tense situations
- An enhanced self-awareness of personal impact upon others, leading to increased self-confidence and hence contributing to an improved ability to work with others in groups and teams
- A developed flexibility in responding to changing situations and adopting a more diverse range of behaviours
- Shared knowledge and learning derived from a wide and diverse range of colleagues; creation of a network of colleagues who can be trusted to support personal learning
- An enhanced ability to communicate with others and to network with them
- Legitimate and protected problem-solving time
- Identification of personal and professional development needs

At the level of the ***organisation*** or ***organisations*** the benefits include:

- An integrated path to personal and organisational learning at as fast a rate as changes taking place in the outside world; this helps to create a learning culture within the organisation or organisations
- Increased political and cultural awareness – enhanced understanding of organisational and professional barriers and how they might be overcome
- Enabling effective action to be taken to resolve difficult issues – to do things differently and to improve continuously; tangible and practical outcomes are produced as a return on the investment of time and finance
- The encouragement of effective teamwork and of inter-departmental, inter-professional and inter-organisational cooperation
- The development of leaders with a flexible and an entrepreneurial or intrapreneurial approach, with an increased readiness to take responsibility and initiative
- Innovative practice as set members work together and discover new ways of achieving results
- A focusing of the energies of committed people
- A complementary and supportive activity to other work-based developmental approaches such as mentoring and coaching

> Doubt ascending speeds wisdom from above.
>
> *(Reg Revans)*

As indicated below in a series of '*vignettes*', at the level of the ***service user***, ***patient*** or ***client outcomes***, action learning has enabled the easier introduction of new clinical, social and community care and managerial procedures; has ensured a more rapid roll-out of new policies; has affected important cost-savings; has increased inter-professional information-sharing; has fostered cross-departmental and cross-organisational working; has improved the clarity of the emerging roles of clinical, social and community care staff; and has initiated the development of educational programmes for both staff and patients/clients/service users.

At the ***societal*** level, what we know about the future is that we do not know much about it! Therefore, the responsibility is not simply to give people tools that may be out-of-date before they have even been fully mastered, but to help them to become confident and competent designers and makers of their own learning tools. In this respect, it has been suggested that action learning can make a significant contribution to the development of social capital. Social capital is collective capacity or efficacy – the quantity and quality of the relational connections within or across any organisation, network or system. It exists in the active connections among people where trust, mutual understanding and shared values make cooperative action and learning possible.

There is also a strong case to be made that action learning can help to make us good citizens of a democracy as it helps us to adopt an active stance to life and helps us to overcome the tendency to think, feel and be passive towards the pressures of life (see Chapter 14).

WHERE IS ACTION LEARNING USED?

From its origins in the UK in the 1960s and 1970s, action learning is now an international phenomenon. It is being used in over 70 member states of the United Nations in Europe, Asia, the Middle East, North, Central and South America, Africa and the Pacific (1,2).

Global corporations make significant use of action learning. The major names include:

AstraZeneca Pharmaceuticals	IBM
AT&T	Marriott
Bayer	Microsoft
British Airways	Motorola
Cathay Pacific	Nokia
Deutsche Bank	Roche Pharma
Exxon	Samsung
Ford Motor Company	Shell
General Electric	Siemens
General Motors	Toyota
Honda	Volvo

While many of these organisations are multi-national corporations where Anglo-American values predominate and action learning seems to *'fit'* well, the existence of national cultures which do not necessarily provide such an easy match has increasingly been recognised (3,4).

The differences between such Western and non-Western cultures have been identified broadly as follows (5):

Western cultures	**Non-Western cultures**
Individualism	Collectivism
Achievement	Modesty
Equality/Egalitarianism	Hierarchy
Winning	Collaboration/Harmony
Guilt (Internal self-control)	Shame (External control)
Pride	Saving face
Respect for results	Respect for status
Respect for competence	Respect for elders
Time is money	Time is life
Action/Doing	Being/Acceptance
Systematic/Mechanistic	Humanistic
Tasks	Relationships/Loyalty
Informality	Formality
Directness/Assertiveness	Indirectness
Future/Change	Past/Tradition
Control	Fate
Specificity/Linearity	Holism
Verbal emphasis	Non-verbal emphasis

Two examples can illustrate this. Many Indonesian organisations are marked by powerfully paternalistic and hierarchical leadership styles, together with such phenomena as '*tepa selira*' (mutual respect) and '*karukunan*' (conflict avoidance) (6) and in Bosnia-Herzegovina (part of Europe but with a strong Asian influence) an action learning set member stated that:

It is good to have knowledge, but dangerous to always show it. (7)

Nonetheless, the continuing spread and popularity of action learning in China (8) and South Korea (9) demonstrate the inherent flexibility of the approach in successfully adapting to different national cultures. This suggests that in non-Western societies action learning needs to be acculturated – that is, conveyed and transferred across cultural boundaries to ensure that its application is user-friendly. This involves adjusting to the particular cultural milieu in order to ensure that the maximum benefits can be realised. This, in turn, requires a keen sensitivity to the underlying assumptions operating in such settings and the resultant ways in which people in such a culture think and act. Acculturation involves attention to such areas as the selection of problems, the composition of the sets, the questioning and reflection process, the commitment to taking action and the nature of facilitation (5).

In the UK, major organisations using action learning include the National Health Service, the BBC, the Civil Service, local government, the John Lewis Partnership and the Police. Other applications take place in a wide range of fields, including social work, the publishing, engineering and construction industries, agriculture, banking, facilities management, community development, teacher education, veterinary science, higher education, the creative industries, passenger transport, small and medium enterprises (SMEs) and an international development and relief agency. The most typical uses of action learning in the UK are as part of an organisation development initiative, for performance improvement and as part of leadership and management development programmes.

WHAT IS THE TRACK RECORD OF ACTION LEARNING IN HEALTH, SOCIAL AND COMMUNITY CARE?

Health care

There is a good case to be made that one of the major roots of action learning lies in health care (10) and within health care in the UK action learning has been applied in the professional fields of nursing, nurse education, midwifery, health promotion, public health, mental health, learning disability and practice development. More generic applications in health care have included multi-agency working, primary care, leadership and management development (especially clinical leadership), clinical governance, information technology and knowledge management.

The most major evaluation ever conducted of action learning in health care was of the early Hospital Internal Communications (HIC) project, which demonstrated that action learning was primarily about organisational change achieved through individual change (11). A more recent health care action learning evaluation study concluded that the learning and development achieved was both specific to the particular issues brought (or surfaced) by the set members and also generic and transferable to other situations. While some of that learning was about growing self-insight, much was also in relation to specific methods and approaches. Both were seen to be sustainable over time and in to other settings (12).

The most recent research on leadership in the NHS concluded that what health care leaders did in practice was relationship-building, negotiating complex cross-boundary activity and exercising political skills. Leaders placed the greatest emphasis on learning from both personal experience and from that of colleagues – which are core to the action learning process (13).

Here are a number of '*vignettes*' – mini-case studies relating to the outcomes of action learning in health care.

- ***Hospital Communications***: In one of the earliest action learning projects (14), Revans worked with a consortium of 10 London hospitals in the 1960s. All the hospitals were experiencing major difficulties in resolving such problems as employee morale, staff turnover and productivity. Revans created sets in which the set members were familiar with the problems, but not with the setting. He established a multi-professional set in each hospital that consisted of a doctor, a nurse, an administrator, a pharmacist and a domestic services manager. Each set, instead of addressing problems in its own hospital, addressed problems in one of the other hospitals, so that each hospital had a set drawn from elsewhere working on their issues. The results were remarkable – reductions in patient stay, improved employee morale, smaller staff turnover and improved communications. When the set members returned to their own hospitals, they took their insights with them and applied them locally. In addition, there was a major improvement in the self-confidence of the set members (11).
- ***Senior Clinical Leaders***: From 2005 to 2017 NHS Scotland's national strategic clinical leadership programme '*Delivering the Future*' used action learning sets as part of a comprehensive programme design, with a particular emphasis on supporting improvement projects as well as personal development and a means of linking theory and practice (15,16). Among the improvement areas addressed have been:
  - Development of a managed health and social care network for older people's services
  - Development of national radiology information to support performance-managed waiting time targets
  - Service redesign from fracture treatment to falls prevention
  - Development of a community dermatology referral management and treatment service
  - Piloting and roll-out of an electronic palliative care summary
- ***Supporting the Nurse and AHP Consultant Role***: An action learning set was formed to support nurse and allied health professions (AHP) consultants already in post. Plymouth University worked in collaboration with NHS Trusts in the South-West of England. Positive outcomes included increased role clarity; improved influencing and negotiating skills; the addressing of issues of work–life balance; reduced professional isolation; the creation of work-plans and the creation of portfolios of evidence (17).
- ***Tissue Viability Best Practice, Hull & East Yorkshire***: A development programme was devised by Hull University for Link Nurse Practitioners (a new role) leading on tissue viability. While there was significant personal development for the programme participants, the organisational outcomes included improved role clarity, the creation of educational programmes for ward-based staff, the development of information aids, care plans and cost-savings achieved from unused and un-required dressings (18).
- ***Point of Care Testing (POCT) Coordinators***: An action learning set made up of the Point of Care Testing Coordinators from each of the acute hospital trusts in the North East of England and Cumbria met on a regular basis for over six years, supported by the North East Pathology Network and the University of Sunderland. The set organised two POCT conferences for health care scientists, developed better understanding of international accreditation standards, developed local standards and created an audit template to self-assess whether such standards were being met (19).
- ***Early Clinical Careers Fellowships for Nurses & Midwives***: This scheme, active since 2007 and aimed at supporting talented nurses and midwives at an early stage in their career to develop personally, professionally and academically, is run by NHS Education for Scotland. Action learning is blended with other approaches, such as Masters-level study,

masterclasses and mentorship/clinical coaching. Fellows have identified action learning-derived outcomes as an awareness of the '*bigger picture*', improvements in their clinical practice, greater personal and professional networking, enhanced personal resilience and increased self-insight, leading to improved self-confidence (20).

- ***Enhancing Compassionate Care***: Funded by Health Education West Midlands and focused on developing a Trust-based approach to the delivery of compassionate care, two action learning sets of ward sisters/charge nurses, supported by Birmingham University's Health Services Management Centre, have devised a programme of work centred on enabling staff teams to support each other in placing compassionate care back at the heart of clinical nursing practice (21).
- ***St. Vincent's University Hospital, Dublin***: The organisational impacts from this project included achieving cost-savings, the introduction of new procedures, the roll-out of new systems and policies, increased information-sharing and enhanced inter-disciplinary and cross-departmental working. Individual impacts included improvements in listening and questioning, improved problem-solving, collaborating and a better understanding of change (22).
- ***Learning Disabilities Rape Victims***: This was part of a project that explored why mainstream rape support services were failing to meet the needs of women with learning disabilities who had been raped. An action learning set brought together women with learning disabilities, representatives from a university, a third-sector organisation and a rape crisis centre. The set enabled them to explore the issues from a range of perspectives, sharing knowledge and expertise and enabling them to begin to develop better service responses. Working together led to a shared understanding of the barriers experienced by women with learning disabilities who had experienced rape and the challenges faced by workers who aim to support them. One output was bespoke easy-to-read information leaflets and relevant training (23).

Social care

While health care has been one of the major proving grounds of action learning, its spread into social care has been slower, despite some early pioneers in the 1990s (24–27). This is somewhat surprising, as it has been noted that action learning has strong links with social work problem solving. There are high levels of risk, uncertainty and change in the public sector generally, and in particular within social work, that require an approach that questions perspectives and assumptions and allows people to feel challenged in a supportive environment as '*comrades in adversity*'. It has been suggested that action learning can support the development of ethical and critical social work practitioners who can support one another in the relative safety of an action learning set (28). In the social work setting, action learning can also support practitioner development, including emotional intelligence, anti-oppressive practice and critical reflection, all of which are desirable for individuals, teams and organisations seeking to keep up with the pace of external change. It is also especially relevant in multi-agency settings where it can help to break down barriers between departments and professions and to foster innovation and inventiveness in practice. Social work also has a person-centred ethos and action learning also adheres to this underlying principle to support each other in times of adversity (28).

The use of action learning in supporting newly qualified social workers (NQSW) has been strongly promoted by Skills for Care – the sector skills council responsible for social care – and by the former College of Social Work. Initially, this was by supporting social care employers firstly through the NQSW Framework for adults' services, and latterly through the Assessed and Supported Year in Employment (ASYE). Many social care employers now use this methodology as part of their '*support package*' for NQSWs, to enhance supervision and reflective practice discussions, to provide additional learning opportunities or as a support for supervisors and managers.

Skills for Care's approach has been to develop a sustainable resource for employers through training action learning facilitators (29). A renewed focus has been thrown on developing reflective and analytical practice and the emphasis has been on developing critically reflective action learning (30).

The potential of action learning for partnership and collaboration between social care and health care was recognised at an early stage by Revans and his collaborators (31–33). Further development often focused on specific areas such as case management (34) or care of the elderly (35). More recently, the importance of inter-organisational work between health and social care has been increasingly recognised as important, as the following vignettes illustrate.

- ***Health and Social Care Partnerships*:** Action learning was used as the keystone of a three-year project jointly funded by NHS Education for Scotland and the Scottish Social Services Council. It involved working with 31 health and social care partnerships with the aim of improving leadership and collaboration in the context of health and social care integration. Significant outcomes included the building of more trustful relationships; a culture change from 'doing to' to 'doing with'; improved medication management and improved understanding and communication across hospital, community, home and social care and general practice as essential elements in progressing partnership working, in order to improve integrated locality working (36).
- ***Multi-agency Public Sector Partnership Teams*:** Action learning sets were formed from management teams of local authorities, the NHS, education and the police with help from the Institute for Local Government Studies at Birmingham University. Issues addressed included hierarchy, power, responsibility and accountability within and between the management teams. The case study concluded that the tensions or 'grit' in such relationships needed to be addressed in order to make progress and that the necessary levels of trust could only be established through set members taking and exploring risks together (37).
- ***Health and Social Care Network in Aberdeenshire*:** A health and social care network of action learning sets comprising general medical practitioners, local social work team managers and social work practitioners was established in eleven areas in Aberdeenshire between 2011 and 2013. One hundred and seventy-two people regularly attended set meetings held over a six-week cycle and created opportunities for constructive challenge and improvement in practice, behaviours and pathways for care of older people with the shared outcome of shifting the balance of care from hospital to community settings (38).
- ***Services for Children and Young People with Learning Disabilities and Difficulties in Yorkshire and Humber*:** Initiated by the former Care Services Improvement Partnership, multi-agency action learning sets across four geographical areas in Yorkshire and Humber met for 12 months in 2007–2008 in order to support service improvements for children and young people with learning disabilities and difficulties and mental health problems. Among the outcomes were the kick-starting of local improvement initiatives, the redesign of client-centred care pathways and the breaking-down of inter-professional and inter-agency barriers (39).

Community care

Delivery of community-based care via a variety of statutory and voluntary organisations builds upon the recognition of a need for effective continuing collaboration between health and social care. Two examples are considered here:

- ***A Multi-Agency OD Programme*:** Stoke-on-Trent City Council planned a management development programme for senior staff, but the consultancy appointed to deliver this managed to convince the local authority that the work should instead be pursued via an Organisation Development (OD) project and should be based around the multi-agency '*umbrella*' of the Local Strategic Partnership – a grouping of public, private, community and voluntary organisations. It involved around 100 '*street-level bureaucrat*' (40) participants drawn from these agencies. A major element of the programme was 10 action learning sets which were based on existing '*area improvement teams*' and focused on problems in local communities such as litter and graffiti, play provision for children and development of a local neighbourhood centre. The sets identified and implemented a range of actions and the initiative also located other issues that had impeded further progress, including staffing churn, different agency cultures, professional languages and levels of commitment and an operational/strategic tension (41).
- ***A Neighbourhood Renewal Programme*:** Brighton University was asked to design and deliver a development programme for people involved in neighbourhood renewal. The '*Action Learning Together*' (ALTogether) programme involved volunteer community leaders, local authority policy-makers, social workers, teachers and residents of the disadvantaged neighbourhood in question. Based around the self-managed action learning approach, the programme was externally evaluated and judged a success (42).

A growing number of examples of such generic inter-organisational working have emerged (43) as well as examples drawn from community regeneration (44), the police (45), the clergy (46) and the voluntary sector (47).

Examination of all these examples drawn from health, social and community care suggests that action learning has:

- Fostered self-awareness, enhanced self-esteem and thus improved self-confidence
- Challenged negative behaviour patterns and routines
- Provided support for those taking on new leadership roles and helped to break down related feelings of isolation and powerlessness
- Firmly rooted leadership development within professional and managerial practice
- Built leadership and innovation across systems, developed effective working relationships and enhanced personal resilience
- Encouraged cross-sector collaborative working and encouraged honest dialogue

REFERENCES

1. M. Marquardt, Action learning around the world in *Action Learning in Practice*, Fourth edition, ed. Mike Pedler (Farnham: Gower Publishing, 2011) 325–337.
2. Y. Boshyk (Ed.), *Action Learning Worldwide: Experiences of Leadership and Organisational Development* (London: Palgrave-Macmillan, 2002).

3. G. Hofstede, *Culture's Consequences: Comparing Values, Behaviours, Institutions and Organisations Across Nations* (London: Sage, 2001).
4. T. Patel, *Cross-Cultural Management: A Transactional Approach* (Abingdon: Routledge, 2014).
5. M. Marquardt, *Action Learning in Action: Transforming Problems and People for World-Class Organisational Learning* (Palo Alto, CA: Davies-Black Publishing, 1999).
6. D. Iriwanto, An analysis of national cultures and leadership practices in Indonesia, *Journal of Diversity Management* 4 (2): 2011: 41–48.
7. J. Edmonstone and J. Robson, Action learning on the edge: Contributing to a masters programme in human resources for health, *Action Learning: Research & Practice* 11 (3); 2014: 361–374.
8. M. Marquardt, Action learning in China, *Action Learning: Research & Practice* 12 (3); 2015: 325–333.
9. Y. Cho and H.-C. Bong, *Trends and Issues in Action Learning Practice: Lessons from South Korea* (Abingdon: Routledge, 2013).
10. C. Brook, The role of the NHS in the development of Revans' action learning: Correspondence and contradiction in action learning development and practice, *Action Learning: Research & Practice* 7 (2); 2010: 181–192.
11. G. Weiland and H. Leigh (Eds.) *Changing Hospitals* (London: Tavistock Publications, 1971).
12. J. Edmonstone and V. Davidson, *An Evaluation of Action Learning Sets Run for The Improvement Network, Trent Strategic Health Authority* (Ripon: MTDS, 2004).
13. Health Services & Delivery Research, *New Evidence on Management and Leadership, Health Services & Delivery Research Programme, National Institute for Health Research* (Southampton: University of Southampton, 2013).
14. R. Revans (Ed.) *Hospitals: Communication, Choice and Change: The Hospital Internal Communications Project Seen from Within* (London: Tavistock Publications, 1972).
15. D. Upton, P. Upton, R. Erol and F. South, *Evaluation of The Impact of Delivering the Future Programmes in Bringing About Improvements in Healthcare in NHS Scotland* (Edinburgh: University of Worcester for NHS Education for Scotland, 2013).
16. J. Edmonstone, The development of strategic clinical leaders in the national health service in Scotland, *Leadership in Health Services* 24 (4); 2011: 337–353.
17. J. Richardson, R. Ainsworth, R. Allison, J. Billyard, R. Corley and J. Viner, Using an action learning set to support the nurse and allied health professional consultant role, *Action Learning: Research & Practice* 5 (1); 2008: 65–77.
18. J. Kellie, E. Henderson, B. Milsom and H. Crawley, Leading change in tissue viability best practice: An action learning programme for link nurse practitioners, *Action Learning: Research & Practice* 7 (2); 2010: 213–219.
19. H. Verrill and A. Parnham, Commissioning point of care testing through action learning, *ACB News, Association for Clinical Biochemistry* 2010: 21–22.
20. A. Machin and P. Pearson, Action learning sets in a nursing and midwifery practice learning context: An evaluation, *Nurse Education in Practice* 14 (4); 2014: 410–416.
21. Y. Sawbridge and A. Hewison, Making compassionate care: The norm starts with our staff, *Health Service Journal* 25 July 2014.
22. L. Doyle, Action learning: Developing leaders and supporting change in a healthcare context, *Action Learning: Research & Practice* 11 (1); 2014: 64–71.
23. A. Olsen and C. Carter, Responding to the needs of people with learning disabilities who have been raped: Co-production in action, *Tizard Learning Disability Review* 21 (1); 2016: 30–38.

24. H. Burgess and S. Jackson, Enquiry and action learning: A new approach to social work education, *Social Work Education* 9 (3); 1990: 3–19.
25. M. Baldwin and H. Burgess, Enquiry and action learning and practice placements, *Social Work Education* 11 (3); 1992: 36–44.
26. T. Morrison, *Staff Supervision in Social Care: An Action Learning Approach* (Harlow: Longman, 1993).
27. I. Taylor, Enquiry and action learning: Empowerment in social work, in *Educating Social Workers in a Changing Policy Context*, eds. M. Preston-Shoot and S. Jackson (London: Whiting & Birch, 1996).
28. C. Abbot and P. Taylor, *Action Learning in Social Work* (London: Sage, 2013).
29. C. Abbott, L. Burtney and C. Wall, Building capacity in social care: An evaluation of a national programme of action learning facilitator development, *Action Learning: Research & Practice* 10 (2); 2013: 168–177.
30. M. Pedler, C. Abbott, C. Brook and J. Burgoyne, *Improving Social Work Practice Through Critically Reflective Action Learning* (Leeds: Skills for Care, 2014).
31. A. Baquer, *Project on Coordination of Services for The Mentally Handicapped* (London: King Edward's Hospital Fund for London, 1972).
32. R. Revans and A. Baquer, *I Thought They Were Supposed to Be Doing That: A Comparative Study of Coordination of Services for The Mentally Handicapped in Seven Local Authorities* (London: The Hospital Centre, 1972).
33. Ali Baquer and Reg Revans, *But Surely That Is Their Job?: A Study in Practical Cooperation Through Action Learning* (Southport: ALP International Ltd, 1973).
34. K. Ball, Action learning: Creating a space for multi-agency reflexivity to complement case management, *Practice* 25 (5); 2013: 335–347.
35. S. Maslin-Prothero, S. Ashby and A. Rout, *Using an Action Learning Research Approach to Evaluate and Develop Inter-Professional Working Among Health and Social Care Staff, Particularly in Relation to The Care of Older People* (Keele: University of Keele, 2007).
36. R. Burgess, Julia Parker and Malcolm Young, *Action Learning Applied in Health and Social Care Partnerships* (Stirling: OLPD, 2014).
37. M. Willis, Tension, risk and conflict: Action learning journeys with four public sector partnership teams, *Action Learning: Research & Practice* 9 (2); 2012: 167–176.
38. www.jitscotland.org.uk/example-of-practice/action-learning-sets/
39. A. Pullen, J. Foster, L. Hall-Bentley, S. Stebbings, S. Tinker and G. Jones, *Working Together to Improve Services for Children and Young People with Learning Disabilities and Difficulties: Summary and Evaluation of An Action Learning Partnership Programme for Service Improvement* (Sheffield: Care Services Improvement Partnership and Yorkshire and Humber Partnership, 2008).
40. M. Lipsky, *Street Level Bureaucracy: Dilemmas of the Individual in Public Services* (New York: Russell Sage Foundation, 1980).
41. J. Edmonstone and H. Flanagan, A flexible friend: Action learning in the context of a multi-agency organisation development programme, *Action Learning: Research & Practice* 4 (2); 2007: 199–209.
42. S. Lawless and A. Penn, *Evaluation of the AL Together Programme: Interim Report* (Brighton: CAG Consultants, 2004).
43. D. Coghlan and P. Coughlan, Developing organisational learning capabilities through inter-organisational action learning. in *Current Topics in Management*, eds. M. Rahim, R. Golembiewski, and K. MacKenzie (New Brunswick, NJ: Transaction, 2002), 7, 24–27.

44. K. Broughton, D. Jarvis and R. Farnell, Using action learning sets for more effective collaboration: The managing complex regeneration programme, *Learning & Teaching in Higher Education* 4 (2); 2010: 16–21.
45. H. David, Action learning for police officers in high crack areas, *Action Learning: Research & Practice* 3 (2); 2006: 189–196.
46. J. Muskett and A. Village, Action learning sets and social capital: Ameliorating the burden of clergy isolation in one rural diocese, *Action Learning: Research & Practice* 13 (3); 2016: 219–234.
47. NACVS Action Learning for Managers: Final Report, Plus Action Learning Matters (Sheffield: National Association of Councils for Voluntary Service, 2004).

PART 2

Practice

PART 2

Practice

5

Preparing for action learning

> If I continue to believe as I have always believed, I will continue to act as I have always acted; And if I continue to act as I have always acted, I will continue to get what I have always got.
>
> *(Marilyn Ferguson)*

ASSESSING THE CLIMATE AND CULTURE

Typically, organisations tend to turn to action learning when:

- They need to tackle difficult problems or to deal with a new and challenging situation
- There is a need to develop leaders and managers who can manage change and uncertainty
- Jobs, roles and organisations are changing
- New partnerships, collaborations and alliances have to be created
- Both personal and organisational development is required
- Traditional, course-based education and training programmes are seen as being inappropriate or ineffective

However, organisations will need to assess exactly how ready they are to embark upon action learning. The extent of organisational readiness will be a significant factor influencing the degree of success of action learning for both individuals and organisations. The organisational setting or context may be more or less conducive to the likelihood of successful outcomes. Readiness is rooted in two questions:

- Does the organisation really want to do it?
- Is the organisation in a place where it is ready to do it?

Ideally an organisation will exhibit a sufficient degree of openness and support to give permission for action learning to develop, while simultaneously providing enough challenge to the status quo to stimulate learning and change. That being the case, it is clear that not all organisations are in such a place. Organisations with a strong '*training*' culture, for example, may not feel comfortable with action learning. Their default tendency would most likely be to constrain uncertainty and aim to establish order through curricula, best practice and set techniques (1). Being in the right place would involve:

- Support and commitment from senior organisational levels
- A willingness to address system-wide issues and to examine *'wicked'* as well as *'tame'* problems (2)
- A tolerance for uncertainty and ambiguity
- An embracing of diversity as a stimulus to creativity
- A degree of discretion and freedom of action for individuals

Assessing whether or not the culture of the organisation(s) concerned is welcoming of action learning can be aided by the use of some helpful tools. The ***Organisational Fitness Ranking*** (3) provides useful questions for consideration by an organisation thinking about embarking on action learning. It directs thinking towards whether action learning should be used to consolidate existing areas of strength or to address areas worthy of attention. It can also usefully identify the different perceptions of various individuals and groups on such matters. The ***Organisational Readiness for Action Learning Questionnaire*** (4) helps an organisation to rate itself against a set of learning organisation criteria and offers a guide to the likely value of action learning. *'Readiness'* is seen as existing when sufficient challenge to the status quo is balanced with an appropriate degree of openness and support. These readiness conditions are often most prevalent early in an organisation's life-cycle because often when organisations mature (become older, larger and more complex) they tend to lose much of this natural learning ability.

More generally, it is possible to identify certain organisational and personal factors which enable or facilitate successful outcomes from action learning – and also others which disable or prevent achievement of such outcomes. They include:

Enablers:

- A close match between the developmental climate of an organisation and the underlying assumptions behind action learning; this also implies a dissatisfaction with the more conventional and didactic approaches to organisational, leadership, management and staff development and with ways of working on complex problems
- A local system that takes a strategic approach to the creation of the action learning sets and links them appropriately to other relevant activities and networks
- Sets being made aware of the wider context within which they are working, including how their organisations work, who and what they need to influence and how best to do this
- An influential person or persons (i.e. a *'champion'*) within the wider system who takes a close and supportive interest, either by design or by adoption, in what sets are doing and who helps them, where appropriate, to grapple with issues
- Sponsors who have either experienced action learning themselves or who fully understand and support the underlying assumptions; this is translated into such actions as prioritising attendance at set meetings over organisational crises and providing the appropriate degree of support and challenge to set members
- Proper account is taken of relevant national policies and issues
- Problems, issues, challenges and questions which the set member works on that are challenging enough
- A set membership that is significantly voluntary and diverse against such criteria as age, gender, geography, organisation, profession, seniority and so on
- Regular attendance of set members at set meetings and follow-through in the workplace on actions agreed in the set meeting
- Preparation for attendance at set meetings – undertaking what was previously agreed and being ready to report on it

- Active and involved participation in set meetings, listening and responding to what is said
- A high level of motivation and a willingness on the part of the set member to take a long hard look at themselves
- A capacity to be open and responsive – willing and also able to open up to others
- A balance between the support and the challenge which each set member receives and also the balance between an emphasis on reflection and on action
- The use of questions in the set which help the set member to address the issue
- These are likely to be open, awareness-raising, elaborating questions and will focus on personal ownership of the issue
- Making the best use of time within the set meeting, so that set members have broadly equal *'airtime'*

Disablers:

- A mismatch between the culture of the organisation and the underlying assumptions behind action learning; this can manifest itself in action learning being adopted, for example, by the Human Resources function but not understood or supported by local management or senior professionals
- Action learning being introduced as an *'island'* activity, disconnected from national policies and issues, local strategic concerns and therefore floating free of the necessary connections within the sets members' contexts
- Non-existence of a senior *'champion'* figure who both understands and supports the purpose and process of action learning
- Sponsoring managers who do not understand action learning, either because they have not experienced it themselves or because their value system is at odds with the underlying assumptions upon which action learning is based; support is therefore typically perfunctory and subject to interruptions by local crises
- Set members who have been *'sent'* to the set as a reward or, more typically, as a punishment, for them to be *'sorted out'*
- An unbalanced set membership, skewed in particular directions, such as professional role and organisation, geographical and gender mix, seniority and so on
- Set members not attending set meetings or turning up infrequently and not following-through on those commitments to action that they have given at those meetings
- Set members not having a relevant and appropriate issue or challenge to bring to the set, or joining the set without it being previously agreed, or bringing something along to the set that they already know how to do
- Passive attendance at set meetings – being there in body but not in mind or feelings
- Non-preparation for set meetings – just turning-up and expecting something to happen, with the onus of responsibility resting on other set members and/or the facilitator
- Set members looking for a *'quick fix'* – a magic bullet which will take care of all of their problems
- Set members with pre-existing and inappropriate mind-sets
- A lack of balance, with too much emphasis in set meetings on either support or challenge or on action or reflection
- Yarn-spinning and using up time in set meetings; hogging the limelight and so dominating the agenda; game-playing and undermining the commitment of others; gossiping and avoiding addressing the real issues

- Giving everyone the benefit of your advice at every opportunity and using the set meeting to score points and show how clever you are
- The use of questions which do not help other set members work on their issue. These can include closed, leading and trick questions and questions can also be poorly timed and overly probing
- Talking about other set members and their problems outside the set

KEY INITIAL QUESTIONS

Organisations considering using action learning will need to ask themselves some key questions, including:

- Will the issues or topics chosen involve all set members in real and significant change?
- Is what is being considered realistic and feasible in terms of the timescale, resources, experience and skills available?
- Are the risks of failure high enough to stimulate action, without being too threatening?
- Are the likely issues unknown enough to need imaginative and creative ways forward?
- Will the issues expose set members to different perspectives and ways of working and learning?
- Are senior people in the organisation really committed to the success of the programme?
- Does the organisation (or organisations) have the power and will to implement changes arising from the action learning process?

TASTER EVENTS

One way of familiarising people with the possibilities of action learning is through *'taster'* events where they can be given a flavour of what it entails. Such a workshop could last one day or half a day and might involve:

- A presentation on the basic concepts underlying action learning
- An opportunity to experience some of the dynamics of a set, possibly through the Slow-Motion Questioning Exercise in Part 3 of this book
- A chance to explore the range of options for future development, including:
  - Intra-organisation or intra-profession sets
  - Multi-organisation and/or multi-professional sets
  - Multi-agency sets
  - Themed sets around a problem, topic or role
  - Kick-start sets, where facilitation is provided only for a limited number of early meetings

There is a paradox here. On the one hand, would-be action learning set members and sponsors need to know enough (in P terms), as early as possible, about action learning in order to make informed choices about whether or not to adopt it, whether to get involved and so on. On the other hand, it is difficult to really understand what is involved in action learning without experiencing it. Therefore, a fine balance between conceptual material and experiential work needs to be struck in such an event.

JOINING AN ACTION LEARNING SET

How might someone go about joining an action learning set?

- The first port of call for a potential action learning set member should be to identify those colleagues and others who have been part of an action learning set and to ask them about their experience. Useful questions to ask them might include:

  How did you become an action learning set member?
  How many meetings did the set hold?
  Over what length of time did the set operate?
  How long did the meetings last?
  Was the set focused on a particular professional or managerial role or on a specific issue?
  Who were the other set members?
  What were the kinds of problems brought to the set meetings?
  What kind of support did you receive from your sponsor or from the organisation more generally?
  How did the facilitator operate?
  What tangible outcomes emerged from the work of the set members?

  This should help to give an impression of what might be involved. However, it would be important to remember that action learning is a very flexible approach and that the experience of one individual (say as part of a business-driven set) might differ from that of another (say as part of a blended action learning programme).
- There would also be value in enquiring whether membership of relevant professional and managerial bodies had a particular view or experience of action learning.
- Useful information might also be available from local Human Resources, leadership development, management development or organisation development specialists who would most likely know where action learning was being used within the organisation or where there might be scope for its adoption. That person should also know about externally based programmes which were either action learning based or included it as a significant part of their design.

> Coming together is the beginning. Keeping together is progress. Working together is success.
>
> *(Henry Ford)*

COMMITMENT

What needs to be clear at an early stage is the level of commitment necessary for success on the part of the set member, but also from their sponsor.

- **Set member:** There are two major areas where set members would need to display their commitment to the action learning process.

  - ***Set meetings***: This involves regular attendance at all the agreed set meetings, preceded by any necessary preparation, and focused on reporting progress in working on the chosen issue. Other set members and the facilitator will ask challenging questions and act, where necessary, as *'devil's advocate'*. It also means agreeing with the other set members the necessary actions to be taken on return to the workplace. There will also be a need to actively listen to the challenging situations of other set members and to support and challenge them as necessary. There may also be informal communication with the other set members, by telephone or email, between set meetings. Regular attendance at set meetings is extremely important, as non-attendance has a negative impact for the non-attending set member but also for the other set members who do attend.
  - ***Workplace***: This is where action on the problem, issue or question takes place, trying-out the ways forward agreed with fellow set members during the set meeting. It also involves reflecting on the success or otherwise of such actions, in preparation for reporting this to the next set meeting.

  It is important to recognise that there are time and energy implications of set membership, but also that the more that an individual invests in the action learning process, then the more powerful the impacts will be, both at the levels of practical action and personal learning.

- **Sponsor/Senior colleague:** There are a number of clear messages that need to be communicated. They are that there will be important pay-offs to you as my sponsor/senior colleague and to the organisation. They will include.
  - A more rapid acceptance of the introduction of new policies and procedures
  - Increased inter-professional and inter-functional information-sharing
  - Greater inter-departmental, inter-professional and inter-organisational teamwork and cooperation, leading to enhanced partnership working
  - Greater role clarity, especially in situations where new roles are created or emerge
- **Organisation:** The key messages that need to be communicated here are that:
  - Perplexing issues, which previously were seen as insoluble, will now be addressed in a much more positive way.
  - Significant organisational challenges will be identified, clarified, addressed and resolved, with tangible outcomes achieved.
  - A culture of continuous improvement will be being generated.
  - Capability will be being built up – the ability to adapt to change, to generate new knowledge and to continue to seek to improve performance.
  - As a result, even in embryo, a learning organisation will be being developed, where the rate of personal and organisational learning is at least as rapid as the rate of change in the world.

In order for this to happen:

- If an individual's membership of the set is part of a wider development programme, then attendance at set meetings may well be compulsory. On the set member's part this will require an openness to try out the approach if they have never experienced it before, even if initially they may feel sceptical and possibly initially reluctant to bring issues to the set.

- The sponsor/senior colleague, may need, depending on the programme, to attend a start-up, mid-point and end-point event, so this may well involve a time commitment on their part.
- The sponsor/senior colleague will need to realise that the set member's involvement in an action learning set will probably be quite unlike their previous participation in any conventional training course.
- The sponsor/senior colleague may need to become a little more well-informed about both the purpose and process of action learning than they have previously been in order to maximise the potential value of the set member's involvement.
- The sponsor/senior colleague will need to work with the set member to identify a real, significant and challenging problem, issue, challenge or question which will involve implementation as well as diagnosis.
- The sponsor/senior colleague may also need to accept that the original or *'presenting'* issue which the set member works on may evolve and that what they start working on may not be what they eventually come to address.
- The sponsor/senior colleague will need to support the set member's regular attendance at set meetings as a worthwhile use of time and an investment for the future for both the organisation and that individual. This may mean seeking to ensure that work crises do not, as far as possible, impinge on the set member's attendance and that it is, in fact, protected time.
- The set member will need to meet with the sponsor/senior colleague regularly between set meetings so that they are up-to-date with what is going on. This will also demonstrate the sponsor/senior colleague's support for the set member's involvement in the set. In those meetings, the set member will need the sponsor's personal support (because sometimes the set member will feel anxious and scared with what they are trying to do) and also their challenge (to put the set member on their mettle, in a helpful way).
- The sponsor/senior colleague may need to accept that what emerges from the set member's involvement in the set might be challenging to both them and to the organisation, as the set member may find themselves questioning some taken-for-granted assumptions.

RESPONSIBILITIES OF STAKEHOLDERS

There is real value in spelling-out, at an early point, the responsibilities of all concerned in the working of action learning. The notion of a *'learning contract'* may therefore be a useful one. The aim should be to avoid a bureaucratic or heavy-handed approach and to emphasise instead a light-touch and minimalist approach.

Nevertheless, it is helpful if it is clear to the set member, sponsor and facilitator exactly what they are signing-up to. An example of such a learning contract might be:

***Set member*:**

- To work with the sponsor to identify and agree an appropriate issue which will be worked on both in and between set meetings, accepting that the issue may evolve or change as the set progresses
- To attend set meetings regularly and to support and challenge fellow set members as they work on their issues and problems
- To listen attentively to other set members, and to be open and generous with questions and constructive ideas
- To follow-up on action agreed at the set meeting back in the workplace and to report on progress at future set meetings

- To respect confidentiality and differences and to be open to learning through action
- To take part in any evaluation activity

***Sponsor*:**

- To identify carefully those individuals for whom participation in an action learning set would be a useful development activity, from the points of view of both the individual and the organisation
- To become as well-informed about the purpose and processes of action learning in general, and of the work of the set member in particular, in order to make informed decisions and choices
- To work with the set member to identify appropriate issues which will be worked on in the set, accepting that these may evolve or change as the set develops
- To support the regular attendance of the set member at set meetings by accepting that set activity is a worthwhile use of time and an investment for the future for both the individual and the organisation
- To help the set member with the implementation of those actions in the workplace that have emerged from set meetings
- To take part in any evaluation activity

***Facilitator*:**

- To model appropriate behaviour, such as high-quality listening skills and asking useful questions, for the set membership
- To be active in the early life of the set in order to foster a sense of collective identity and mutual interdependence amongst set members
- Thereafter, to be timely and appropriate in interventions in the set's life, concentrating largely on the process, that is, how set members and the set as a whole is working – with the aim of enabling individual and group learning to take place
- To encourage set members to focus on agreed actions
- To take part in any evaluation activity

PROBLEMS, PROJECTS, TOPICS, ISSUES, CONCERNS, CHALLENGES AND QUESTIONS

Man can learn nothing except by going from the known to the unknown.

(Claude Bernard)

All these words are used, often interchangeably, to characterise the particular focus of the work of the set member. The lack of a single and precise definition is quite deliberate. Some people, for example, dislike the use of the term *'problem'* and others, at the outset, may have only a fairly *'fuzzy'* understanding of what the specific issue or concern might be. For some set members, the idea of calling it a *'project'*, for example, can potentially feel constraining as they can feel quite hemmed-in by what they consider a *'project'* to be, based upon prior experience, and so feel unable to explore other possible avenues of learning. Whatever it is called, it will be the vehicle for action and learning so it must be demanding without being overwhelming. It must address an unresolved issue at some level and may well seem intractable in nature, at least at the outset. In effect, it is a *'social laboratory'* in which real-time change occurs and, as such, no-one can ever be fully prepared for what may emerge.

The progenitor of action learning, Professor Reg Revans, identified what he called the *'risk imperative'* that an action learning project should embody. Set members work from a basis of ignorance and confusion on an issue which carries a major risk of a penalty for failure. Unless the set member feels the risk, and is aware of what is being risked, then learning is unlikely to happen. If there is no risk, then consequently there is no significant learning. People may see change as being positive when it involves others, but not necessarily when it means that they, too, must think and act differently. Profound self-review and subsequent self-development come from acting on a problem which carries a real possibility of failure. Set members may fear, and sometimes encounter, consequences for the risks that they take. When the organisational culture is not supportive of mistakes, then there can be more pressure to perform than to learn. In spite of what they might espouse, senior management may *'punish'* people who question too much or suggest ways forward that are not aligned with the dominant organisational culture. This is why action learning projects place such a strong emphasis on moving beyond diagnosis to action in the workplace.

> Why not go out on a limb? That's where the fruit is.
>
> *(Will Rogers)*

In considering what issue to tackle, it is important that:

- ***It should matter***: The issue to be worked on should be real and important to the organisation and to the individual and certainly not be a contrived exercise. This implies that there should always be an identified sponsor associated with the issue who will support the set member who is working on it. The key stakeholder or stakeholders concerned need to really care about the issue in question. Failure to address the issue would be likely, in time, to provoke a crisis of some kind. Ideally, therefore, the issue should be critical and urgent and should trouble and/or excite the set member. It has to be something which a set member can *'get their teeth into'* and in which they feel *'I am part of the problem and the problem is part of me.'* In other words, addressing the issue should make a real difference.
- ***It should be practical:*** It should be based, as far as possible, on data and the outcome should produce ground-level consequences – in other words, a tangible effect. This means the set member will be involved in the often infinitely messier business of action (implementation) as well as diagnosis. This may have implications for the timescale associated with the problem as action learning programmes are often time-limited and this period of time may not always match the realistic timescale for action on the issue. The issue chosen should either lie within the set member's sphere of influence or they should be given the necessary authority required in order to carry matters to a conclusion.
- ***It should be challenging***: It should be *'hurting'* and the status quo should therefore not be an option. If a set member could simply progress the issue on their own, is absolutely clear about what should happen next and has the necessary will to take matters forward, then they would have little need for the set's support and challenge. The issue chosen could therefore potentially be something entirely new, but should be something which the set member has not previously addressed, and which they want to be able to progress.

- ***It should add value***: The outcome should benefit both the organisation and the set member in some way or another.
- ***It should connect***: It should build on, or take account of, the existing organisational structures and culture – it must take notice of what is realistic and possible.
- ***It should be complex in nature***: It should deal with issues which extend across various parts of an organisation or even across several organisations.
- ***It should be capable of being learned from***: The issue should not be so specialised or obtuse that other set members feel unable to challenge or to support the set member who brings it. Set members should be able to explain the issue to others and to report-back at set meetings on progress (action) and personal insight (learning).
- ***There should be no expert solution available***: The topic chosen should have no obvious *'right'* answers.
- ***It should not be too large***: It is easy to take on an issue which is overwhelming and so to become frustrated at the lack of progress. Judgement about the duration of the entire sequence of set meetings and the time available within each should therefore influence the choice. Ideally, the issue addressed would be current over the anticipated life-span of the set, although as previously noted this is not always feasible.
- ***It should be defined in some way***: The issues chosen are likely to range along a continuum from tightly focused to loosely focused. Tightly focused issues will be defined in terms of the time and other resources available to address them or in the light of the abilities and learning needs of the set members to address them. An example might be the merging of two departments or functions within a defined time period. Loosely focused issues can often be helpful to set members, particularly if they come from a particular professional background with a related mind-set which encourages them to consistently see problems in a particular way. The more loosely focused and open-ended the issue, then the more the set member may be inclined to cope with a range of different perspectives and to learn to live with a greater degree of ambiguity than before, thus preparing them for future challenges. A loosely focused issue might, for example, be an exploration of the possible provision of a new or extended service to clients. Whatever the style of definition, all set members will need to address such basic questions as *'Whose problem is this?'*, *'Why is it seen as a problem?'* and *'Is the problem, as presented, symptomatic of something deeper?'*

> You must do the thing you think you cannot do.
>
> *(Eleanor Roosevelt)*

Organisational problems, challenges, issues and questions come in a wide range of shapes and sizes. Revans distinguished between what he called *'puzzles'* and *'problems'*. The former were like crossword puzzles and had *'best'* solutions and *'right'* and *'wrong'* answers. They were *'difficulties from which escapes are thought to be known'* - organisational embarrassments which could be resolved by the application of P alone. Examples might be the technical process of performing heart surgery – it is complicated, but there is a known process for doing it – or writing a business case for a service within a tightly structured organisation where there is highly specific guidance, a standardised format and clearly defined parameters. He contrasted this with *'problems'* – complex, rather than complicated; dynamic, rather than static; novel or even recalcitrant and intractable. This distinction maps very neatly onto another very useful distinction which can be made between *'tame'* and *'wicked'* problems or issues (2).

Tame (or benign) problems (Revans' puzzles):

- Can be described by a fairly clear and simple statement
- Exist where the degree of uncertainty which is associated with the problem or issue is limited
- Are where the root causes of the problem or issue are either already known or are relatively easily discoverable
- There is broad agreement between all interested parties about what *'success'* would look like
- Are constant and do not fundamentally change over the passage of time
- Respond to the well-known tools of rational planning and management
- Are marked by the fact that previous experience and practice with the same or similar problems are useful guides towards a solution
- Have definitive and optimal solutions which would apply in any setting or context – and are therefore transferable
- Have a clear *'stopping point'* so that it is understood when a solution has been reached
- Can be objectively evaluated

Tame in this context does not necessarily mean simple – a tame problem or issue may be very complicated technically. Tame problems are typically operational problems, concerned with organisational efficiency, with looking *'inwards and downwards'* and focusing on issues of control and performance. The issues are usually immediate and short-term and emphasise the maintenance of consistency and correction of deviations from required targets or standards.

Wicked problems (Revans' problems):

- Are characterised by a high degree of uncertainty
- Interact with other problems and so cannot simply be addressed in isolation
- Will appear *'fuzzy'* – that is, incomplete, possibly contradictory and often unclear
- Sit outside single professional and managerial hierarchies and exist across organisational boundaries
- Defy rational analysis and planning
- There will be multiple perspectives on what exactly the issue is and what the right way forward might be
- Are strongly related to the particular context within which they exist
- Previous experience and practice appear to be of little help towards any resolution
- Progress will require both individuals and organisations to change their mind-sets and their behaviour – to learn new ways of working and to choose between contradictory values
- What exactly *'success'* in addressing the issue might be is difficult to define
- Resolution of the issue may even, in turn, create further problematic issues

Examples of wicked problems or issues would include childhood obesity, urban planning, homelessness, neighbourhood crime, alcohol and drug addiction, child abuse and communication issues between health and social care professionals. Wicked problems are usually also strategic problems – located between day-to-day operational challenges and overall policy direction and concerned with developing a sense of coherence and with fostering a sense of direction and purpose. Typically, wicked problems are hard to describe and defy the *'rational'* analysis associated with tame problems, not least because, due to complex interdependencies, actions taken towards resolution often tend to lead to unintended consequences. As a result, they may seldom be completely *'solved'* but rather they change shape and/or lead into other, related problems. They also often require collaboration between different agencies, all of who have a stake in such problems.

> Some problems are so complex that you have to be highly intelligent and well-informed just to be undecided about them.
>
> *(Laurence J. Peter)*

There may be a tendency within health, social and community care to either assume that all problems or challenges are tame in nature or to pretend that what are actually wicked problems are in fact tame, and therefore amenable to being worked-on by rational analysis and planning. It has been suggested that, especially in health and social care:

> Our learnt instinct...is to troubleshoot and to fix things – in essence to break down the ambiguity, to resolve any paradox, to achieve more certainty and agreement and to move into the simple system zone. (5)

Action learning is very capable of addressing both tame and wicked issues. In the case of the former, tangible and concrete outcomes can be quite easily identified and achieved. In the case of the latter, the diversity of set membership, the asking of powerful and penetrating questions and the challenge which the process entails, all mean that action learning is particularly suited to addressing such issues (6–8). It is also important to remember that all problems or issues will have a dual public and private nature. Addressing an issue successfully will involve internal (private) changes in people as well as external (public) changes in the organisation. What is happening here is a reframing of the problem at both personal and system levels.

> There are dreams of love, life and adventure in all of us. But we are also sadly filled with reasons why we shouldn't try. These reasons seem to protect us, but in truth they imprison us. They hold life at a distance. Life will be over sooner than we think. If we have bikes to ride and people to love, now is the time.
>
> *(Elizabeth Kubler-Ross)*

Problems familiar and unfamiliar

Figure 5.1 illustrates that problems can be considered as a combination of familiar and unfamiliar tasks and familiar and unfamiliar settings. Figure 5.1 contains four cells:

***Cell 1*:** Here someone remains within their present job and addresses a familiar issue. The continuing danger here is that what has been chosen may either be only a tame issue or *'puzzle'* or that it has been contrived and therefore does not embody the degree of challenge required.

***Cell 2*:** Here a person remains in their current job but tackles an issue which they have never previously addressed within that work role – something both novel and challenging.

***Cell 3*:** Here someone takes on an issue with which they have previously had some success in their current job, but now they are faced with the challenge of trying to address this earlier success by tackling the same issue in another department, function or organisation where they are unfamiliar with the history, culture and ways of working.

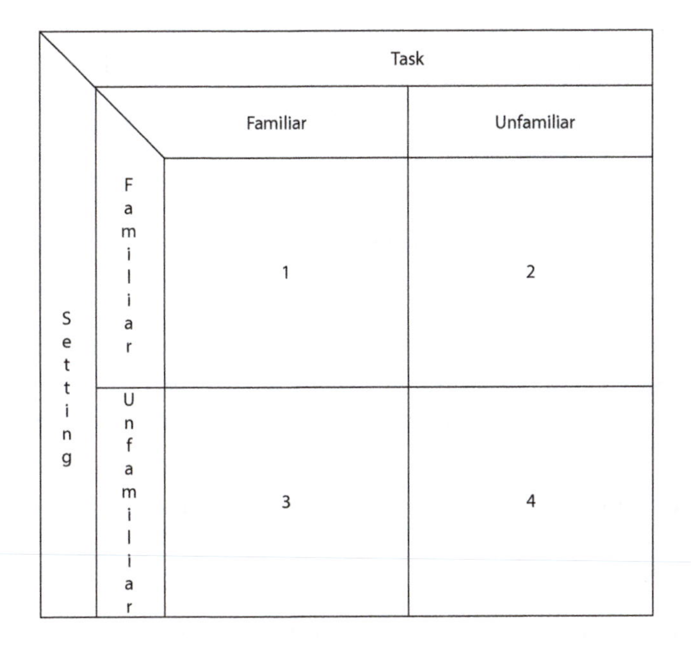

Figure 5.1 Problems familiar and unfamiliar.

Cell 4: Here someone moves to another organisation or an unfamiliar part of their own organisation and tackles an unusual and previously unfamiliar problem. While most action learning problems recently addressed tend to be in Cells 1 and 2, there is a powerful case to be made for Cell 4 projects, especially if the aim is to take the set member out of their comfort zone and be placed in a situation where they must ask fresh questions and challenge their own long-held assumptions.

A problem shared is a problem halved.

(Anon)

Problem-solving inputs

Action learning is about both the development of people and the addressing of problems in work organisations. It has been suggested (9) that there are two major inputs required for a problem-solving process to be successful. They are:

- ***Hard (or technical) inputs***: These are about problem resolution, task achievement, efficient resource-use, attention to the bottom line and the meeting of deadlines, targets and objectives. They emphasise the need to be logical, rational, quantifying and structuring, and are expressed in constructive challenge and debate.
- ***Soft (or socio-emotional) inputs***: These relate to personal feelings, motivations and drives. They emphasise the importance of relationships and the need for a secure and safe setting and peer support, where personal experience can be reviewed and re-interpreted.

These two inputs are complementary and cannot, and should not, be separated from one another – and in action learning they are not, as Figure 5.2. shows.

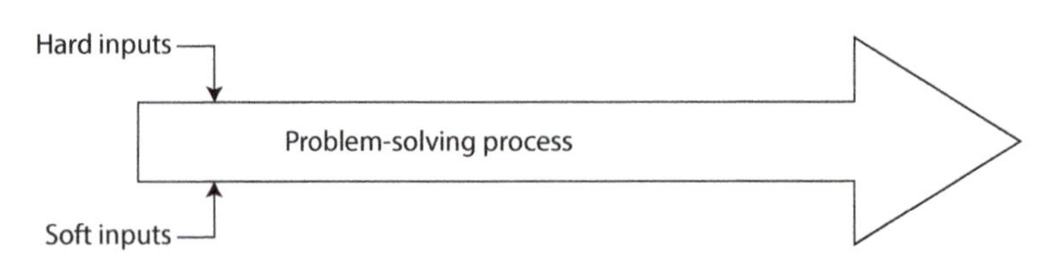

Figure 5.2 Inputs to the problem-solving process.

Biases

In tackling personal and organisational difficulties, most people, for most of the time, tend to rely on a set of heuristic principles or rules of thumb, in order to simplify matters (10). The most common rules of thumb are:

- ***Recent and past occurrence***: The tendency is to assume that what people remember happened in the recent past is most likely to happen again in the future.
- ***Representativeness***: This tendency is to assess the likelihood of an occurrence by matching it with a pre-existing category or stereotype.
- ***Anchoring and adjustment***: Choices are not made in a vacuum. People typically start with some underlying basic assumptions and different individual's different assumptions lead to different personal choices.

Within the context of an action learning set the set members will inevitably bring these rules of thumb with them – but the questioning nature of the set will mean that they will be subject to challenge and may need to revise them as a result.

> There are more problems than answers
> Pictures in my mind that will not show
> There are more problems than answers
> And the more I find out the less I know
>
> *(Johnny Nash)*

REFERENCES

1. M. Pedler and C. Abbott, *Facilitating Action Learning: A Practitioner's Guide* (Maidenhead: McGraw-Hill/Open University Press, 2013).
2. H. Rittel and M. Webber, Dilemmas in a general theory of planning, *Policy Sciences* 4; 1973: 155–169.
3. M. Pedler, *Action Learning for Managers*, Second edition (Aldershot: Gower Publishing, 2008).
4. M. Pedler and K. Aspinwall, *Perfect Plc?: The Purpose and Practice of Organisational Learning* (Maidenhead: McGraw-Hill, 1996).
5. P. Plsek and T. Greenhalgh, The challenge of complexity in health care, *British Medical Journal* 323 (7313); 2001; 625–658.
6. J. Edmonstone, On the nature of problems in action learning, *Action Learning: Research & Practice* 11 (1) (2014) 25–41.

7. L. Crul, Solving wicked problems through action learning 2014, *Action Learning: Research & Practice* 11(2); 2014: 215–224.
8. K. Grint, Wicked problems and clumsy solutions: The role of leadership, *Clinical Leader* 1 (1); 2008: 54–68.
9. B. Garratt, *The Learning Organisation* (London: Fontana-Collins, 1987).
10. A. Tversky and D. Kahneman, Judgement under uncertainty: Heuristics and biases, *Science* 185 (4157); 1974; 1124–1131.

6

Action learning sets

We must indeed all hang together or, most assuredly, we shall all hang separately.

(Benjamin Franklin)

Action learning sets are the means by which set members work out and pursue their own actions in the workplace and learn from that experience through processes of review, reflection and planning ahead. They are concerned with:

- Helping set members to learn from the issues which they are addressing, so that they increasingly challenge their own and others' assumptions
- Diagnosing the nature of the problem and then, most importantly, going on to implement practical ways forward
- Moving into '*uncharted territory*' where the issues are unfamiliar, rather than areas where set members already have experience

Sets can be of two types – the stranger set and the in-house set. In the **stranger set** the set members do not come from the same workplace. It is therefore correspondingly easier to facilitate because set members are not involved in each other's organisations and are thus better able to offer disinterested listening. The **in-house set** is more problematic and involves more risks, but the potential pay-off is possibly greater. The likely dangers are that the set may prefer and resort to general discussion (as a means of '*learning inaction*' or avoiding the surfacing and addressing of major issues in their organisation) and that set members' previous knowledge of a situation or a group or an individual being described may increase a tendency to be judgemental.

SET FORMATION

The formation of sets is a vital process and there are a number of ways in which sets can be formed. The major criteria are:

- ***Interest:*** Involvement in a set should, wherever and whenever possible, be voluntary because the personal motivation of set members is hugely powerful in sustaining their effort over the life of the set.

- ***Level of challenge*:** This should be broadly similar for all the set members.
- ***Mix of professional roles and organisations*:** This is in order to ensure a diversity of experience and background and to promote the potential for cross-system learning and networking.
- ***Common areas of interest for addressing similar challenges*:** This, however, may also limit the possible scope for learning.
- ***Diversity of personal style*:** A '*rich mixture*' can be created by the personal skills of set members, together with their professional and organisational experiences and styles. Sufficient contrast is needed to provide the '*grit in the oyster*', although too great a diversity may make it difficult to develop a shared sense of identity. Diversity needs to be balanced with equality. See also Chapter 7 on the Energy Investment Model.
- ***Equality*:** It is helpful if the set shares a broadly common age range or work experience, together with broadly the same level of responsibility, career progression and achievement, although this can be difficult to achieve. No one set member should feel out of their depth. Where an in-house set is used, line managers should probably not be in the same set as their subordinates, particularly where there are dominant personalities and the set members come from a status-driven and hierarchical organisational setting.
- ***Gender mix*:** A balance, as far as is possible, of male and female set members.
- ***Geography*:** For logistical travel and meeting purposes.
- ***No personal animosity*:** Action learning is not intended as a means of conflict resolution, so those with a '*history*' between them would most likely not feel safe in one another's company, would be less likely to open up and would colour the overall tone in a negative manner for the other set members.

Sets can be formed around a specific need, such as people entering a new role or tackling a new initiative, and this particular approach is straightforward and easily managed, but potentially may remove the element of choice on the part of potential set members and may also lessen the degree of diversity and '*stretch*' available.

SELF-SELECTION OF SET MEMBERSHIP

This is a process for forming sets out of a larger group such as members of a development programme and relies upon an iterative means to arrive at flexible criteria for self-selection of set members. Clear ground rules for pursuing this process are needed and these are:

- All sets must be **finally** formed at the same time.
- Conversations all take place in one room with everyone taking part.
- Sets need to be formed by the end of an agreed time period.

People must consider their own criteria for forming or joining a potential set and will need to engage in dialogue with other potential set members. A series of conversations in pairs, trios and larger groups across the agreed time-period can lead to a more '*natural*' emergence of sets. The facilitator can help this process by suggesting questions which might be addressed, such as:

'Do I want to work with people I already know?' 'Why is this?'
'Should I aim to join a set with people I've never met?' 'Why is this?'
'Should I consider the professions or organisations of the others?' 'Why is this?'

'Should I aim to work with someone whose behaviour I find challenging?' 'What are the advantages and disadvantages of doing this?'
'Who will really challenge me?' 'Why do I want this?'
'Does my issue have any implications for my choice?' 'Why is this?'

This approach enables people to create their own learning environment from the outset. It does take time and may possibly provoke feelings of anxiety and uncertainty for some – the age-old feeling of '*Will I be picked for the team?*'. Nonetheless, the pay-off lies in the sense of ownership which set members then have in relation to the set which they opt to be a member of.

ALTERNATIVE SET GROUPINGS

Sets comprise around a maximum of seven or eight people. There are three alternative configurations for set groupings:

- ***Horizontal sets*:** These are sets made up of people working at a similar organisational grade or status level within one, or across several, organisations. This is the configuration adopted by most sets. Shared experience and common ground help to reduce barriers and to encourage greater levels of trust. However, if set members' perspectives are so familiar to each other it may be difficult to challenge shared views.
- ***Vertical sets*:** These are sets made up of members drawn from different levels within the same profession or function. They illustrate a high level of support and commitment from the profession or function concerned and promote the concept of equality of contribution from all individuals. They allow a full spectrum of views on particular issues and provide a ready-made means of communication between all the levels concerned, so enhancing the likelihood of subsequent action. However, if there are over-hierarchical or dominant relationships already in existence then this grouping may stifle set members' input and create difficulties for them in communicating ideas and concerns.
- ***Hybrid sets*:** When there are a number of sets running across an organisation or organisations there may be an advantage in also creating another set made up of representative members of the '*regular*' sets in order to focus on what continuing learning is being achieved across the whole system, rather than only the specific issues which set members are addressing.

QUESTIONS REGARDING SET MEMBERSHIP

There are some useful questions worth asking by organisations and by facilitators when considering the potential set membership. They include:

Is there anyone missing from the proposed membership who could really contribute to the life of the set?
Will every set member be allowed to attend set meetings or will they be subject to pressure from their boss and/or colleagues for doing so?
Will the proposed configurations produce all-female, all-male or mixed gender sets and if so does it matter?
What will be the maximum and minimum number of set members for the set to work effectively?

The answers to these questions will vary according to the focus of the sets, the organisational setting and the overall intentions in using action learning.

AGREEING SET GROUND RULES

Early in the set's life it will be important to establish ground rules to guide and govern the behaviour of the set members and the facilitator; to allay any fears about what might happen in the set and to model a shared responsibility between the set members and the facilitator. Such a code of conduct makes it less likely that set members will be disappointed or frustrated by the behaviour of other members.

Ground rules are of two types:

Practical ground rules: Cover such matters as:

- ***Attendance and punctuality***: The importance of being there (attendance) and being there on time (punctuality)
- ***The life-expectancy of the set***: Over what period of time is it intended that it will meet?
- ***The frequency and duration of set meetings***: How often will the set meet and for how long on each occasion? Will there be breaks (e.g. for holidays) and if so, how many and when?
- ***The format of meetings and how time will be allocated within them***
- ***Whether and how notes will be taken to record specific actions arising from each meeting***
- ***Declarations of any conflicts of interest***
- ***Exchange of contact details***: To enable contact by set members between set meetings

Behavioural ground rules: These would address such matters as:

- ***Commitment and priority***: Set members are busy people with many calls on their time. Attending set meetings takes a degree of commitment, as does pursuing the workplace-based activity that occurs between meetings. Self-discipline on the part of set members will therefore be necessary and this needs to be considered at the outset.
- ***Confidentiality***: The '*personal*' stays in the room. All set members are likely to subscribe to this in principle, but it will be important to specify exactly what this entails in practice. Confidentiality can never be absolute, so agreeing on limits and when and how information might be communicated outside the set will be important. Clarity in this area allows each set member to make an informed choice about what to disclose in the set meetings. For example:
  - Should confidentiality extend to discussions involving any third parties mentioned during the meetings?
  - Should the identity of individuals or organisations mentioned in set meetings be disclosable to other parties without their permission?
  - In what circumstances can set members and the facilitator communicate information to people outside the set?
- ***Respect***: For other set member's views, which means being non-judgmental.
- ***Timekeeping***: To ensure that each set member has a fair share of time available for their issue, it will be important to keep to both the external time boundaries of the meeting (so starting and finishing on time) as well as the internal time boundaries (the time allocated for each set member).
- ***Equal airtime***: Roughly equal time allocation for each set member carries with it the implication that other set members are there to listen and then to enable the focal set member to work on the issue they are tackling. Should a set member not be getting the

kind of help which they need then they should feel totally OK to say so. It is important to avoid the use of personal anecdotes, so possible danger signs might be hearing comments such as:

> We all know what he's like – his reputation goes before him. Let me tell you about …
> I've had a similar problem with my staff – here's how I sorted it.
> I had difficulties with her when she worked for me. Let me tell you about it.

- ***One person speaks at a time*:** There should be no talking-over or interrupting the contributions of other set members. The '*space*' belongs to the set member presenting a question or issue and any personal material belonging to other set members should be rigorously excluded from that space.
- ***'I' language*:** Set members need to always say '*I*' rather than '*one*', '*we*', '*they*' or '*you*' when they mean '*I*'. This, although simple to state, is often quite hard to achieve in practice.
- ***'And' rather than 'but'*:** When disagreeing with another set member it is helpful to begin a sentence with '*and*', rather than '*but*', as this illustrates that two divergent views can co-exist without one seeking to demolish the other. Once again, this is challenging to achieve in practice.
- ***No 'shoulds' and 'oughts'*:** There is a powerful tendency for set members to use words such as '*should*', '*shouldn't*', '*ought*', '*oughtn't*', '*must*' and '*mustn't*'. These are effectively commands, and should therefore be avoided.
- ***Clarity*:** It should be OK to check out assumptions that appear to be being made and to ask questions if something said by a set member is not understood.
- ***Allow silence*:** This gives other people, especially the focal set member, time to think and also conveys the sense that they are actually being listened to.
- ***Encourage expression of feelings about the problem*:** Feelings are facts too.
- ***The right to say*** '*No*' or to decline to respond to a question or a challenge.

The exact number of ground rules adopted is not important and will vary from set to set. It is better to establish five ground rules that people will stick to rather than 25 that they ignore. The most important ground rule to establish is that all ground rules are open to renegotiation and that new ground rules can be agreed at any time that the set feels it is necessary.

LOCATION AND VENUE OF SET MEETINGS

This will clearly depend upon geographical travel distances and times for set members. A quiet, adequately heated and well-ventilated comfortable room is the basic requirement, with comfortable chairs, preferably of the same design and arranged in a circle or rectangle. Access for the less able should be considered at the outset, as should transport and/or parking facilities. Refreshment and meal arrangements must be clear and flipcharts, pens, paper and so on easily available.

There should be no interruptions or distractions. A single '*neutral*' venue might be chosen or alternatively the set members might take it in turns to host set meetings.

In considering the venue of set meetings, the issue of boundary protection is important. This means ensuring that set members feel that they are operating in a private, safe and supportive environment where they can feel OK about addressing their work-related concerns. The set acts as a holding environment or transitional space in which set members can handle their anxiety, so the extent to which the set is able to exclude the immediate demands and pressures of the set members' work environments and to create a space which is truly the set's own for the duration of the set meeting, without any interruptions or intrusion of work pressures, is likely to be a major key to success.

FREQUENCY OF SET MEETINGS

Sets need time in order to work properly and this will vary depending on the set and the needs of its members. Because of the cycle of action and reflection, sets feed on the work that goes on between the set meetings. So the life of the set depends to a major extent upon the issues that individual set members bring to the set meetings.

Sets typically run for periods of 6–12 months, but there does need to be a clearly defined end-point. The gap between meetings should not be so close that attendance and time are problematic, nor so far apart that momentum, a sense of continuity, mutual confidence and trust are lost. Meetings need to be planned and booked well in advance and key holiday dates and work pressure '*peak periods*' should be taken into account in order to ensure maximum attendance.

DURATION OF SET MEETINGS

The larger the set membership, the longer meetings need to last. A set should, as a rule of thumb, allow at least 45 minutes per participant at each meeting, and there may be value in adding a further 30 minutes to the overall time for slippage or comfort breaks. While no set is typical, a meeting involving five members might last for three to four hours but a meeting involving seven or eight members would most likely last a whole day.

WHAT HAPPENS IN THE SET

Set meetings typically move through a number of stages:

- '***What's on Top***': This involves set members checking-in with each other, catching-up with where they are at personally and sharing any immediate '*hot*' news. This helps to reintroduce and reintegrate the set and to reconfirm the group identity, while keeping the set rooted in workplace realities. Sometimes a warm-up exercise might be used for the same purpose, particularly in the early days of the set's life (see Part 3 of this book for examples).
- ***Agenda-setting***: This may involve confirming what was agreed at the previous meeting. In other cases, set members will agree on an agenda and running order and structure the time available. The basic premise that all set members have equal airtime might be modified, by agreement, depending on particular need or urgency.
- ***Progress-reporting***: Set members take it in turns to report on the current state of play with regard to their issue since the last meeting. Preparation pre-meeting by set members helps to structure time well within their '*slot*'; it also helps to develop clarity about what they want to focus on and to lay the ground for identifying the necessary next actions. Set members bring the totality of themselves to the process and can explore as much as they feel comfortable with, while experiencing both support and challenge from other set members. Set members have a range of options for how they might use their time slot. They might, for example:

- Ask the other set members to listen while they give a short presentation and then ask for comments. They might have a pre-prepared flipchart or handout listing the key points that they want to address, or present them on a flipchart in real time. If they do this, they then talk, without interruption, for as long as they wish, about the situation, but leaving sufficient time for questions and comments from other set members.
- Ask for questions from the other set members which are designed to help the individual concerned to come to a deeper understanding of their issue.
- Ask the other set members to brainstorm ways of tackling a problem which they currently face.
- Request the other set members to discuss the question they have presented while:
  - They themselves take personal notes of useful ideas that may emerge
  - Tape-record their time slot and replay it later
  - Review and record options, then decide on action

For each set member's '*slot*' there are effectively three stages which are gone through:

- ***Divergence***: An opening-up of the issue; the asking of questions regarding the context; who are the key people who are involved?; what has happened before?; and what specifically is it regarding the issue that is of concern?
- ***Consolidation***: Clarifying and testing-out explanations regarding the issue. This can involve reconsidering, re-conceptualising, re-ordering or re-framing the issue.
- ***Convergence***: This involves narrowing down the choice of possible ways forward and asking the set member what they intend to do next.

The set meeting thus focuses on each set member and their issue in turn, supporting, challenging and questioning – and also offering resources of various kinds – contacts, sources, materials and so on, with set members helping the person with the issue to learn from what has happened and to find a way forward. People bring the whole of themselves to the process of the set and have the freedom to explore as much as they feel comfortable with, without making a rigid boundary between work and non-work issues.

The tacit knowledge of each set member mentioned in Chapter 1 becomes more explicit through the social interaction that takes place within the set because the environment in which this dialogue takes place powerfully influences the ability of the set members to exchange and develop their mutual understanding. They increasingly modify their perspectives and so make sense of their worlds through this social engagement.

As the set progresses, the balance of time devoted to different activities changes. Time spent on describing or reporting on the issue declines, as does time spent on clarifying it; that is, the nature and background of the issue, the range of options available and so on. With the passage of time, more and more time is devoted to attempts at resolution of the problem and to the practical actions in the workplace that are required.

> Every truth passes through three phases. First, it is ridiculed. Second, it is violently opposed. Third, it is accepted as being self-evident.
>
> *(Arthur Schopenhauer)*

- ***Review***: At the end of each set meeting, some time for reflection, feedback and discussion on individual and group processes is valuable as a means of monitoring the effectiveness of the set, concentrating on such questions as:

  What worked well today?
  What was difficult today?
  Was there any problem with this meeting, and if so, what was it?
  Do we need to do something differently in future?
  How can we be more effective next time?

TIME AND PROCESS

Set members usually come to set meetings from a work environment where the default position is to '*shoot from the hip*'; to troubleshoot and to fix things quickly – to achieve greater certainty and agreement and to be seduced by instant solutions. To this can also be added the often-frenzied intensity and repetitiveness of daily work events. The dominant questions faced by set members in such contexts are:

> What worked before that we can use?
> How quickly can we arrive at a decision?
> How much can we get done?
> Sleep faster – we need the pillows!
>
> *(Polish saying)*

Ambiguity and paradox are therefore avoided in favour of certainty, with a preference for instant solutions and an overwhelming '*bias for action*' (1). This is grounded in:

- ***The felt urgency of the task***: An all-pervading culture of targets and deadlines limits the time available for any comprehensive exploration of issues and reduces the willingness to be reflective.
- ***Avoidance of reflection***: Taking problems only at face value avoids the possibility that they might be highly complex.
- ***Avoidance of decisions***: If a possible decision is deemed risky and the work environment does not support learning from experience then the outcome is often risk-averse behaviour and decision avoidance – the arena of the '*definite maybe*'.

By contrast, dialogue in the set involves slowing down, listening and reflecting and this can be extremely liberating for some, but correspondingly difficult for others who may seek to change the tempo of the set to match that of their work environment.

Some set members may therefore feel uncomfortable because it takes time and practice to unlock the ability to reflect. It may feel extremely awkward – like a right-handed person trying to sign their name with their left hand.

It is really important to emphasise that action learning fosters **dialogue**, rather than debate or discussion. The origin of the word '*debate*' means to '*beat down*'. The word '*discussion*' has the same root as '*percussion*' and '*concussion*' and emphasises analysis, breaking-up or breaking-down and different viewpoints. A discussion is like a game of table tennis, with people batting ideas around in order to win a game. The rule is to follow the topic under discussion. The word '*dialogue*', on the other hand, comes from the Greek '*dia-logos*' meaning to '*hang from*'. A dialogue emphasises the idea that meaning can flow between people and lead to a greater and shared understanding. It is best understood as an exchange of speaking and listening which is directed not at proving one right and another wrong, but more of a process of exploration or joint inquiry. Through dialogue hidden assumptions are articulated, newer and deeper appreciations are gained and unseen possibilities are surfaced. Through being a witness to, and a participant in, a shared conversation, people can see different perspectives and connections and achieve insights that are simply not possible on their own.

Dialogue is therefore about emergence – the bringing forth of new and previously hidden meanings and understandings – less pre-planned and more spontaneous.

Emergence will happen only if the initial conditions (embodied in the set ground rules) are right; if the interactions are self-referential and reinforcing, and if the interactions enable feedback to be given (2). This distinction between dialogue and debate is important – in action learning dialogue offers a chance to respect, question, consider and apply different contributions by allowing them time to '*hang*'.

Argument and debate (the beating-down of ideas), by contrast, allows little time or respect for others and has a competitive edge – coming up with the '*best*' idea or '*trumping*' another's contribution.

> It's not that I'm so smart, it's just that I stay with problems longer.
>
> *(Albert Einstein)*

RESISTANCE TO LEARNING

Some individuals tend to develop resistance to learning, as it involves personal change and challenges or replaces their existing view of themselves and of the world.

Action learning involves surrendering a degree of stability in order to embrace something new and uncertain, so it is perhaps not surprising that such resistance can be triggered. This can relate, for example, to:

- A dissonance between the action learning approach and more traditional educational approaches with which set members may be much more familiar. The seeming lack of structure and the focus on collective learning may potentially generate an initial feeling of confusion and conflict (3).
- The process of questioning deeply rooted values and assumptions can be disturbing for some, as individuals question some of those beliefs that have governed much of their lives and careers. The longer an individual has followed a taken-for-granted belief, then the more difficult it is likely to be to change that belief (4). For some individuals, the gulf which they experience between their own perspective and other realities might provoke such strong feelings of uncertainty, fear or frustration that it might interfere with their reflection process and so lead to resistance (5,6).
- Group dynamics within the set itself. The degree of diversity in set membership can be experienced as '*difficult and discomforting*' (7) and different levels of hierarchy can also potentially exist within sets (8).

Such resistance needs to be recognised as a possible response by some set members and should be addressed by the set members and by the facilitator. The set holds the set member's uncertainty until they can manage it for themselves. It acts as an intermediate and transitional arena which makes room for the feelings and emotions of all set members, as well as their rational calculations, to enable what may potentially be unique to emerge, rather than slipping into well-meaning but premature understandings and solutions that avoid discomfort and effort. Learning in this way, with others, obviously involves vulnerability and risk-taking by individual set members as they admit to the limits of their understanding or even to their lack of understanding. The antidote to this vulnerability is the atmosphere of trust created in the set, such that individuals may feel psychologically safe to both unlearn and learn (9). Trust, in turn, develops a sense of empathy – the ability to stand in another's shoes, to feel with them and not just for them. The development of trust and empathy takes time and the iterative nature of set meetings serves to foster both (10). Trust and empathy emerge from the combination of support and challenge.

SUPPORT AND CHALLENGE

Central to all set meetings are the twin activities of support (*'emotional warmth'*) and challenge (*'light'*). Support cannot simply be engineered but takes some time to build. An appropriate degree of support is often needed before any real challenge can be acceptable. Warmth therefore comes before light. Support comes through active listening and the asking of questions that help an exploration of the issues involved and the possible different angles to consider them. In asking such questions a key internal consideration is *'Is what I am about to say going to be helpful to that person?'*

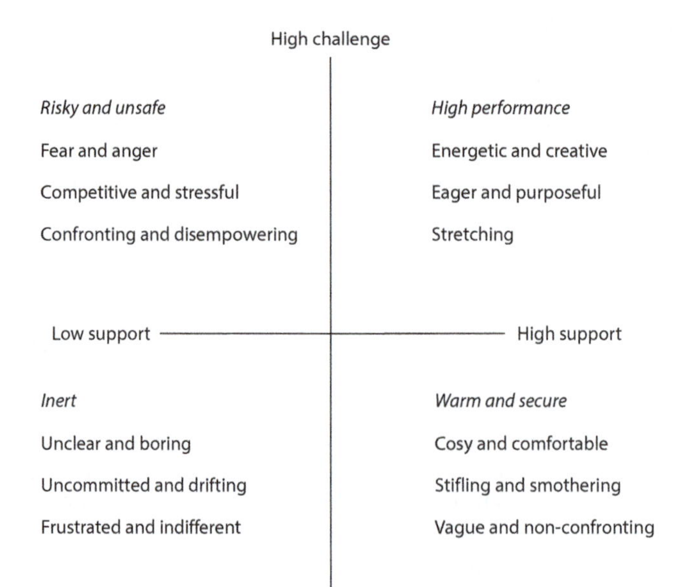

Figure 6.1 Support and challenge.

Challenge is to assumptions, to perspectives and to mind-sets – often playing the role of devil's advocate and asking uncomfortable '*What if?*' questions. Such challenge is not aggressive, but is intended to support personal resolution into action and to ensure that the actions chosen have been reflected on adequately. Too much challenge, too early, is often experienced as being stressful and counterproductive, but too little challenge is also unhelpful. Balancing support and challenge helps the learning process, as shown in Figure 6.1.

Appropriate behaviour in sets therefore involves:

- ***Concern for the well-being of other set members***: This means being committed to being an active set member and being prepared to collaborate with others. All set members need to care sufficiently about their colleagues to want them to succeed with their issue and to learn from the experience.
- ***Empathy***: Empathy is the understanding of the role, context and emotional state of set members. It is not about:
  - Giving advice
  - Giving an evaluation
  - Making a judgement
  - Giving an interpretation
  - Making a challenge

The deeper and fuller is each set member's understanding of their fellow set member's situation, then the more they will be able to find a form of words to enable them to move forward. It involves supporting and challenging as seems necessary and continually asking the question of one's self '*Is this helpful?*'. This also means a willingness to share in the feelings and thoughts of someone else – to ask yourself 'What does it feel like to be ***that*** person with ***that*** *problem?*' – an attitude which is both thoughtful and curious about the person with the problem – a kind of '*intelligent naivety*'.

- ***Each set member as the expert on their own issue***: The person asking the question or addressing the issue will always have access to information which they might not, either by choice or circumstance, share with other set members. Giving the set member *an* answer will probably not be the answer that is most relevant and appropriate to the situation that the set member finds themselves in. So only by believing that people can help themselves, can effective help be given. Respect is therefore needed for the judgement of other set members in identifying exactly what they do and do not choose to share in the set's discussion. In practice, therefore, this involves allowing each set member to present their issue in their own way and avoiding passing judgement or offering solutions. It also means active listening, not talking over or interrupting, and allowing others plenty of time to reflect.
- ***An action focus***: Always taking the actions agreed at the set meeting back in the workplace. In order to get the most from action learning set members do need to undertake preparation for set meetings – most importantly to take the actions which they agreed at the previous meeting. Useful questions for set members to ask in preparation include:

  What have I done since the last meeting?
  What are the outstanding action points, and why?
  Do I still see the issue in the same light as I did originally?

> What have I learned so far from what I have done – about the issue, about myself and about others?
> What are my next steps likely to be?
> What do I need from the next set meeting?
> How might the other set members help me?
> Trust arrives on foot and leaves on horseback.
>
> *(Dutch proverb)*

LEAVING A SET

Sometimes a set member will decide to leave the set. This may be due to a number of reasons – a change of job, problems with home or work circumstances or a feeling that action learning is simply not for them. A set member deciding to leave needs to let the set know in advance and to advise the other set members and the facilitator of their reasons. This gives the whole set time to work through the valuable process of leave-taking.

Experience can be a very '*slippery*' teacher. For most people and for much of the time little is actually learned from experience. Action learning seeks to throw a net around slippery experiences and to capture them as learning, by encouraging reflection, promoting insightful inquiry and leaving responsibility for action firmly with each set member.

> The minute you supply a person with the answers, by that very action you block them once and for all from the opportunity of inventing these same answers for themselves.
>
> If you want to go on an ego trip, to show how smart you are, give the answers. But if what you want is action to be taken then you must refrain from giving the answers.
>
> *(E.M. Goldratt)*

REFERENCES

1. R. Harrison, Choosing the depth of organisational intervention, in *The Collected Paper of Roger Harrison*, ed. Roger Harrison (New York, NY: McGraw-Hill, 1995), 13–32.
2. A. Battram, *Navigating Complexity: The Essential Guide to Complexity Theory in Business and Management* (London: The Industrial Society, 1998).
3. H. Platzer, D. Blake and D. Ashford, Barriers to learning from reflection: a study of the use of groupwork with post-registration nurses, *Journal of Advanced Nursing* 31 (2); 2000: 1001–1008.
4. J. Mezirow, *A Guide to Transformative and Emancipatory Learning* (San Francisco, CA: Jossey-Bass, 1990).
5. S. Brookfield, *Developing Critical Thinkers: Challenging Adults to Explore Alternative Ways of Thinking and Acting* (Buckingham: Open University Press, 1987).
6. K. Trehan and C. Rigg, Beware the unbottled genie: unspoken aspects of critical self-reflection, in *Critical Thinking in Human Resource Development*, eds. C. Elliot and S. Turnbull (London: Routledge: 2005), 11–25.

7. M. Reynolds and K. Trehan, Learning from difference? *Management Learning* 34 (2); 2003: 163–180.
8. A. Yeadon-Lea, Action learning: the possibility of differing hierarchies in learning sets, *Action Learning: Research & Practice* 10 (1); 2013: 39–53.
9. D. Coghlan and C. Rigg, Action learning as praxis in learning and changing, *Research in Organisational Change and Development* 8; 2012: 59–89.
10. J. Edmonstone, Action learning, performativity and negative capability, *Action Learning: Research & Practice* 13 (2); 2016: 139–147.

7

The energy investment model and action learning*

Action learning set members bring to their membership of the set a combination of energy and attitude, and this produces identifiable styles of behaviour, rather than types of people. Everyone has different levels of energy and different states of mind at different times and our behaviour always has an impact on others as a result. How people behave and feel is, however, at least partly under their own control or influence (1), but this can be difficult at times. Everyone gets the most from any experience if their personal energy is high and if their attitudes are positive, but if individuals cannot achieve this then potentially it creates difficulties for the rest of the set membership.

Figure 7.1 shows two dimensions – **energy**, which can be high or low; and **attitude**, which can be positive or negative. This creates four cells in the matrix – Spectator, Victim, Cynic and Player.

SPECTATORS

Spectators have a positive attitude but low energy and tend to feel:

- Positive about what is happening and want to contribute
- Anxious and lacking in confidence
- Reluctant to get involved in the work of the set
- Threatened when too exposed by the set's workings
- Reluctant to take risks
- Most comfortable when *'watching on the sidelines'*

They tend to react by:

- Acknowledging the good ideas of others but being reluctant to change themselves
- Working harder than ever at their own previously successful behaviour
- Avoiding taking undue risks
- Trying to *'ride things out'* until things return to normal
- Keeping a low profile

* An earlier version of this chapter appeared as 'Learning and development in action learning: The energy investment model', *Industrial and Commercial Training* 35 (1); 2003: 26–28.

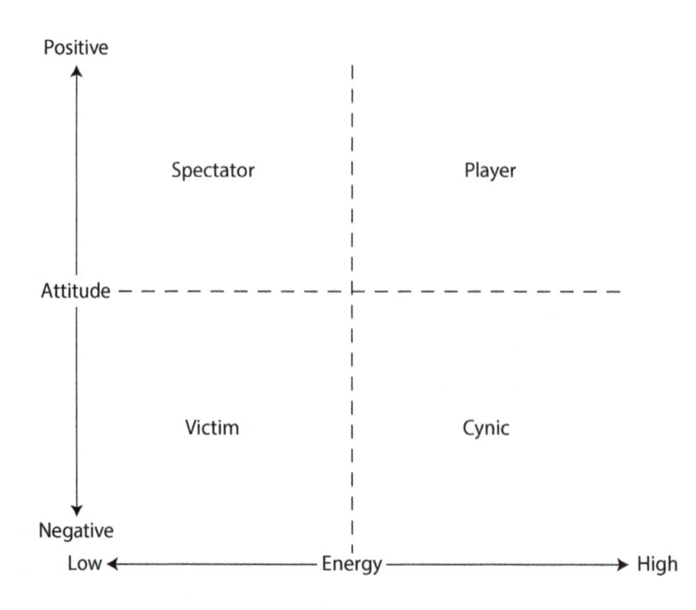

Figure 7.1 Energy investment model.

The kind of support which Spectators need includes:

- Understanding and help in coping with their fear and lack of confidence
- Effective role models
- Plenty of feedback, encouragement and positive reinforcement from other set members
- Stretching, but achievable challenges, both in terms of the issue on which they are working and in relation to the behaviour of their fellow set members

The kind of questions which will stimulate Spectator set members include:

Why do you think this might not apply to you?
Who will do this for you if you don't do it for yourself?
How could you justify leaving this to others?
What's stopping you from having a go?
Can you afford to miss this opportunity?

VICTIMS

Victim set members have a negative attitude and low energy. They tend to have bruised self-esteem and to feel:

- Unhappy or depressed
- Overwhelmed by work
- Powerless and fearful of mistakes

They tend to react both at work and in set meetings by:

- Blocking out challenges
- Avoiding confronting issues

- Retreating into safety
- Avoiding risk and doing the minimum necessary
- Avoiding thinking about what might happen

The support Victim set members need includes:

- Understanding and help in dealing with their stress and frustration
- Peer encouragement
- A series of mini-challenges and successes to rebuild their confidence – fellow set members can help their colleagues to *'eat the elephant a spoonful at a time'*

Useful questions for Victim set members include:

Do you really want to feel like this?
How much can you get back in control?
Who might help you to get back in control?
What could you do to make a start?
What is the worst thing that could possibly happen if you tried something new?

CYNICS

Cynic set members have high energy but a negative attitude and tend to feel:

- Not listened to at work (and so also potentially by their fellow set members) and thus excluded and constrained
- Rebellious and determined to block any change which they do not personally own
- Surprised at the stress felt by others
- That they are *'right'* – and angry at the world for ignoring them
- Frustrated by what they see as other people's confusion and whinging
- Overly confident in their own ability

They tend to react by:

- Expressing their frustration over the pain and hesitancy displayed by others
- Arguing against changes and always seeing the negatives
- Pressing for quick solutions and for decisive actions – and then criticising them!
- Being oblivious to the consequences of their negativity on others
- Bringing both Victims and Spectators round to their own perspective

The support which Cynic set members need includes:

- Humouring – but only to a point
- To be given a chance to take personal responsibility for their actions
- Pairing with a Player set member
- Being confronted about the negative aspects of their behaviour
- Reminding about what the set or the project or issue is actually for
- Clear ground rules and boundaries

Helpful questions for Cynic set members include:

How much do you know about the impact that you have on others?
What happened to make you feel this way?
Could you see things differently?
Could you get a better return on your efforts? How might you do that?
Would there be a better time to do this?

PLAYERS

Players have a positive attitude and high energy and so make excellent set members.
They typically feel:

- Challenged and stretched by both the issue on which they are working and by interaction with other set members
- Comfortable with the need to change
- Open to possibilities and ideas and to suggestions about these made by other set members
- Optimistic about the longer-term future
- In control of their own destiny
- Not afraid of short-term mistakes and setbacks

They tend to react by:

- Seeking the longer-term silver lining behind the short-term dark clouds
- Viewing ambiguity and change as challenge and opportunity
- Finding humour in a range of different situations and using it as a tool in their interactions with others
- Treating life as a whole (and not just their work on their issue or the set itself) as a continual learning experience
- Expanding their personal comfort zone

Player set members need:

- Reward and support from their peers for being key people in change and transition
- Flexible personal growth opportunities coupled with tangible and visible rewards
- Latitude to *'do it their way'* and to model this effective behaviour to others
- Support from others when they take a stand against a Cynic set member
- Respect, recognition and thanks from their colleagues in the set
- Not to have all the work of the set *'dumped'* on them

Useful questions for Player set members include:

Are you taking others along with you or are you too far ahead of the pack?
Might others see you as chameleon-like – or as flip and shallow?
How sensitive are you to the fear of change in others?
Is your optimism with regard to the future really well-founded or not?

This energy investment model can be useful for both set members and the facilitator, as a means of identifying exactly where individual set members appear to be and what might be needed in order to move them forward.

> On the basis of avoided tests, people conclude that constraints exist in the environment and that limits exist in their repertoire of responses. Inaction is justified by the implantation, in fantasy, of constraints and barriers that make action "impossible." These constraints, barriers and prohibitions then become prominent "things" in the environment. They also become self-imposed restrictions on the options that managers consider and exercise when confronted with problems. Finally, these presumed constraints, when breached by someone who is more doubting, naïve or uninformed, often generate sizeable advantages for the breacher.
>
> *(Karl Weick)*

REFERENCE

1. D. Goleman, *Emotional Intelligence: Why It Can Matter More Than IQ* (London: Bloomsbury Publishing, 1996).

8

The key skills

ACTIVE LISTENING

> When you talk, you are only repeating what you already know. But if you listen, you may learn something new.
>
> *(Dalai Lama)*

Active listening to other set members allows each person to learn about that person's needs and wants; to understand better what motivates them and what makes them feel valued – and so serves to build the necessary trust and empathy. The aim is to allow each set member to express themselves as fully and as openly as possible; to help them to '*think out loud*' while working on their issue and to be sympathetically heard and understood. There are four elements to active listening:

- ***Listening***: This involves listening with real attention in order to try and understand the thoughts and feelings of the other person – and why they think and feel the way that they do, without wanting to change them in any way. It is the:

  > ability of the listener to capture and understand the messages communicated by the presenter, whether these messages are transmitted verbally or non-verbally, clearly or vaguely. (1)

  Listening can focus on the set member's ***thinking*** (i.e. what thoughts, assumptions and judgements lie behind the words?), their ***feelings*** (also behind the words in relation to where the set member is now or at the time being spoken of) and their ***intentions*** (listening to what the set member intends to do or their commitment to any intended actions).

  Some hints for effective active listening include:

  - Everyone has two ears and one mouth and they should be used in that proportion.
  - As far as possible, it is important to face the set member who is talking with an upright posture that conveys attention by looking interested and staying alert.
  - This means an open posture because crossed arms and legs may convey, to the focal set member, a closed stance. Maintenance of eye contact is also important.

  - Minimising distractions. Don't fidget or play with pens or mobile phones. It is OK to make notes if there is a need to remember something and it does show interest, provided that it does not significantly interrupt eye contact.
  - Aiming to stop internal '*self-talk*' in seeking to pay attention to the focal set member. Try repeating what the set member is saying in your mind a fraction of a second after they say it. Do not try and plan what you intend to say next.
  - Checking out with yourself whether the speaking set member is triggering any internal feelings and memories that are more yours than theirs. If they are, try not to react to them.
  - Attending to more than just the set member's words – taking note of the language used, the tone of voice and their body language.
  - Don't leap in with personal anecdotes regarding similar experiences, but listen without interruption and take your cue from the set member before intervening.
  - Leave pauses and allow for silence. While many people can feel embarrassed and uncomfortable with this and so seek to fill the silence with words, the set member may need time to reflect internally and privately – important information often comes as an afterthought, so it is unwise to finish people's sentences for them.
- ***Paraphrasing back***: It is important to use at least some of the focal set member's own words in order to let them know that you have actually heard them, as sometimes people can be quite surprised about exactly what they have said – so reflecting it back to them can potentially be very powerful.
- ***Checking understanding***: Do not automatically assume that you have understood what the set member has said, because it is very easy and tempting to impose your own frame of reference. So, for example, if they say '*I feel bad*', then you could say '*Bad about what?*'
- ***Suspending judgement***: Every set member has a reason for their particular perspective and are most likely personally motivated to work things out and to move things forward. They are therefore quite capable of addressing their problems, given the time and the space to think things through. So do not jump in to '*fix*' problems – it is quite disrespectful and disempowering and you are most likely doing it for your own benefit than for theirs.

Active listening can, however, be hampered by:

- ***Evaluative listening***: When we impose our own values on another set member's message and judge what we hear while it is being communicated instead of putting our thoughts to one side to hear what is truly being said.
- ***Comparison***: When we are making comparisons between ourselves and what the set member is saying.
- ***Inattentive listening***: When we are distracted by other things, such as our own emotions or by, for example, tiredness.
- ***Rehearsing***: Someone who is preoccupied with their own response to what a set member is saying probably is stopping listening and attending to that person.
- ***Second-guessing***: Simply not allowing the set member who is speaking to tell the story at their own pace.
- ***Listening with sympathy, rather than empathy***: By offering sympathy at feelings of loss or of sorrow we may get in the way of helping a set member to move on. Empathy is the

ability to observe and not absorb, so that we can respond authentically and not simply react to the other.

Listen, or your tongue will make you deaf.

(Native American proverb)

QUESTIONING

'Forty-two!' yelled Loonquawl. 'Is that all you've got to show from seven and a half million years' work?' 'I checked it thoroughly,' said the computer, 'and that quite definitely is the answer. I think the problem is, to be quite honest with you, is that you've never really known what the question is. Once you know what the question is, you'll know what the answer means.'

(Douglas Adams – The Hitchhikers Guide to The Galaxy)

Insightful questioning grows directly out of active listening. The quality of the questions asked is a function of our ability to listen effectively. Questions seek to enable a set member to broaden or deepen their view of the issue they are addressing and to take responsibility for themselves in order to work it through, rather than being given '*solutions*' by others. Good questions come from a deep interest in the set member's experience and provide them with the opportunity to ponder further.

The American social scientist, Chris Argyris, identified two behaviour models which have direct relevance to questioning (2). They were:

***Model 1*:**

- Asking questions in such a way as to get the other person to agree with one's view
- Advocating one's own view in a manner that limits others' questioning of it
- Privately evaluating the other person's view and attributing causes to it

***Model 2*:**

- Actively inquiring into the other person's views and the reasoning that supports them
- Advocating one's own view and reasoning in such a way that encourages others to challenge or confront it and to help me discover where my view may be mistaken
- Stating publicly the inferences that one makes about others and the data that lead to those inferences, and inviting others to correct those inferences if indeed they are inaccurate

Action learning sets create the opportunity to practice Model 2 behaviour.

The instigator of action learning, Reg Revans, suggested that there were three major questions that every set member needed to pose in relation to their issue. They were:

- ***Who knows?*** Who has useful information? Who has the facts, concepts, arguments, ideas and principles that will determine the dimensions of the problem and not simply official policies, opinions, half-truths or personal views?

- ***Who cares?*** Who has the emotional investment and energy to mobilise change? Who is involved and committed to an outcome, rather than who just simply talks about the issue? The phrase '*When all is said and done, more is said than done*' is pertinent here.
- ***Who can?*** Who has the power and influence to allocate or reallocate resources so that change can happen? Who, when faced with the facts, commitment and energy, has the ability to say '*Yes*'? Who can establish and sustain a momentum for change?

Such questions relate to three crucial processes in human action – ***thinking*** (Who knows?), ***feeling*** (Who cares?) and ***willing*** (Who can?). Educational institutions tend primarily to concentrate on the first question to the detriment of the other two because it is the process which most people are familiar, but which leads to the danger of '*paralysis by analysis*' where diagnosis and planning seldom lead on to action. The degree of emotional commitment (feeling) and power (willing) that exist are also important in ensuring that things actually do happen.

Set members may sometimes need assistance in translating the issue they want to address into a challenge, so there is often a need to move from a focus on the complex nature of the problem itself into one where the focus is '*How can I .... ?*' So particularly at the outset of an action learning project further useful questions to consider are:

- ***What is it that you do?*** What is the nature of your work, role or task?
- ***What are you trying to do?*** What exactly is driving you? What is your motivation?
- ***What is it that is stopping you?*** What are the blockages or obstructions getting in the way?
- ***Who and what can help you?*** What are the resources that you need to draw upon or mobilise?

The intention is always to find and use questions which encourage set members to question themselves, so a good question is ultimately selfless. It is not asked in order to highlight how clever the questioner is nor to generate ever more information for the questioner. Rather, it is a way of opening-up the set member's own view of their issue.

> The idea was fantastically, wildly improbable. But like most fantastically, wildly improbable idea it was at least as worthy of consideration as a more mundane one to which the facts had been strenuously bent to fit.
>
> *(Douglas Adams)*

So, questions from set members and the facilitator can really be helpful and can cover a range of options:

- ***Open questions*:** These are aimed at stimulating an extended free response and are questions that begin with '*Who?*', '*What*', '*Where*', '*Which*', '*Why*', '*When*' and '*How*'.
- ***Specification questions*:** These aim to elicit more detail about the problem situation and could include '*What exactly is the issue?*', '*What do you want to achieve?* ','*How would you know if you had achieved it?* ', '*How important is that to you on a 1–10 scale?*' and '*Everyone?*'
- ***Justifying questions*:** These provide an opportunity for the set member to further explain their reasons, attitudes or feelings and might include '*What assumptions might you be making here?*', '*How would you explain that to someone else?*' or '*Could you help me to understand you by putting it another way?*'

- ***Elaborating questions***: These give the set member an opportunity to expand on what they have already begun to describe. Examples include '*What exactly happened?*', '*Could you say a little more about that?*', '*And then what happened?*' or '*Can you elaborate on what you have just said?*'
- ***Personal ownership questions***: These imply not only that the set member has a responsibility for owning the issue, but also for making those choices that contribute to moving it forward. Examples include '*So, who owns this issue?*', '*How much energy do you really have to tackle this?*', '*What's preventing you from acting?*', '*How do you see your own behaviour possibly contributing to this situation?*' and '*Are there ways in which you might be helping yourself more?*'
- ***Awareness-raising questions***: Such questions encourage self-awareness on the part of the set member and focus on positive ideas for future action. They might include '*How did you feel when you were involved in that?*' or '*What do you imagine it would look like if you did it differently?*'
- ***Focusing on feelings questions***: These aim to tease out the emotions linked to the issue in question. Such questions are best posed tentatively as the set member should know their own feelings better than anyone else. Examples might be '*How do you feel about that?*', '*Deep down, what do you really want?*', '*Are you really being honest with yourself here?*', '*What excites you the most?*' and '*What worries you the most?*'
- ***Hypothetical questions***: These pose a situation or a suggestion – a '*What if … ?*' or '*How about … ?*' and can be useful for introducing a new idea or challenging a response. Some examples here might include '*If you were advising yourself, what exactly would you say?*', '*If you were told that your future job prospects depended on changing the way you worked, what would you do first?*', '*If you were in charge, what would you tackle first and how would you go about it?*' and '*If things were exactly right for you in this situation, how would they have changed?*'.
- ***Checking questions***: These check what the questioner is hearing or correct their understanding. They might include '*What have you already tried?*', '*What are your options for action here?*' or '*Is this always true in every situation?*'

> 'Why?' and 'How?' are words so important that they cannot be too often used.
>
> *(Napoleon Bonaparte)*

In contrast, there are unhelpful questions and these include:

- ***Closed questions***: These can only be answered by a '*Yes*' or a '*No*' and this curtails the set member's options for responding. Often they begin with '*Do you …. ?*', '*Are you …. ?*' or '*Have you …. ?*'. Occasionally they can have a more positive use when they can be used as a challenge, such as '*Do you really want to do anything about this?*'
- ***Leading (or loaded) questions***: These put the answer into the set member's mouth and typically demonstrate that the questioner already knows (or thinks that they know) the answer.
- ***Multiple questions***: This involves rolling several questions into one with the result that the set member is probably going to be confused and is inevitably likely to choose the easiest question and so avoid the difficult one that might be part of the same '*package*'.
- ***Long-winded questions***: These will probably be misunderstood. The most powerful questions are usually between seven and ten words long.

- ***Overly-probing questions*:** These are questions that the set member is not yet ready to answer, given the current level of trust in the set.
- ***Poorly-timed questions*:** These interrupt the set member from working on the issue themselves and arrive at an inappropriate point in the helping process.
- ***Trick questions*:** These are likely to cause resentment, de-motivation and even withdrawal.
- ***Too many questions*:** This might feel like an interrogation and lead to defensiveness.

> The 'silly' question is the first intimation of some totally new development.
>
> *(A.N. Whitehead)*

GIVING AND GETTING FEEDBACK (3)

It is inevitable that as part of what happens in an action learning set that set members will both give and get feedback on their behaviour in the set and also as a reflection on what activities they report on in a work context. Feedback is a powerful process from which set members can understand better the impact of their own behaviour. It is a way of helping them to refine that behaviour, can help to clarify their identity and be used to uncover underlying beliefs. It is also one of the most effective ways of inviting other set members to change their behaviour.

Feedback says as much about the person giving it as the person receiving it. It is useful, therefore, to see it as a conversation to uncover, as far as possible, the impact of behaviour in order for someone to decide whether or not they want to change that behaviour.

While most set members are likely to be reasonably eloquent and fluent, feedback is a focused activity and not to be confused with criticism or praise. Feedback is specific, descriptive and clear, rather than general, judgemental, personal and blaming. Therefore, good feedback should be:

- ***Owned*:** All feedback should be owned by the person giving it and so should be couched in '*You–I*' statements, such as '*When you .... I felt ....* '. A description of someone's behaviour would be followed by a statement about the impact of that behaviour, such as '*When you banged your fist on the table it made me feel anxious.*'
- ***Descriptive, not evaluative*:** Good feedback is only offered on specific observable behaviours – unambiguous descriptions of words said or actions taken, rather than on supposed mental states or personality. The focus is on the behaviour – what someone does – rather than on the person – what someone might imagine that person is. It means acting as a mirror and not a judge, by helping someone to see themselves more objectively and unemotionally, instead of creating defensiveness by sitting in judgement on them. It implies the use of adverbs (which refer to actions), rather than adjectives (which refer to qualities). It frequently begins with such phrases as '*When you did ....*' or '*When you said ....*'. It is crucial to leave out interpretations. For example, rather than '*When you were angry....*' (which is an assumption or interpretation of what was behind the action), it would be important to say '*When you banged your fist on the table ...*'.
- ***Directed*:** Good feedback should be focused on behaviour that the set member can do something about. It means emphasising what someone could do differently instead of simply saying what has been done poorly. Such criticism without specific suggestions for improvement simply creates frustration and defensiveness without helping the set member to improve. For example, if a set member is committed to their current job, but

is describing a life and/or career predicament which they find themselves in, a fellow set member might ask '*Have you even thought about leaving?*'

- ***Balanced***: Good feedback considers the needs of the receiver as well as those of the giver. It will be destructive if it is given because of the giver's needs to say something and without consideration of the person receiving the comments. Feedback is as much about behaviours that had a positive impact as on those that did not. So, for example, a set member might say '*When you winked at me I felt that you understood exactly what I was saying.*'
- ***Well timed***: Feedback should be delivered in a timely way – at the earliest opportunity and as close to the situation which is being described as possible, rather than being saved to be delivered later (a '*cashing-in of vouchers*') –but also depending on the set member's readiness to hear it. Excellent feedback delivered at an inappropriate time may do more harm than good.
- ***Specific, not general or abstract***: For a set member to be told that they are '*dominating*' will probably be less useful than being told '*When this point was being discussed I felt that you did not really listen to what other people said and I felt forced to accept your argument or be attacked by you.*' It is also important to avoid evaluating ('*You were so good at presenting your issue*'), making generalisations ('*You always* ...' or '*You never* ....') or using abstractions ('*You are so devious* ...'). Feedback is more meaningful if reference is best made to the here-and-now rather than the from-time-to-time.
- ***Solicited***: Feedback is much better if it is asked for rather than imposed and if there is a resulting degree of self-review. It is an offer, not an imposition, a revenge or a punishment.
- ***Communicated clearly***: Thinking about what to say and the way it needs to be said, in advance, is helpful, so that what is heard by the set member is what the person giving feedback intended.
- ***In appropriate amounts***: Rather than storing-up material in order to feed it back, it is better to deliver feedback in '*digestible*' amounts. Focusing on the amount of feedback that the set member is likely to be able to use is more helpful than focusing on the amount that the giver has and might like to impart. It is intended to help the recipient and not to satisfy the giver's needs.
- ***Explore alternatives, rather than give solutions***: Doing this shares responsibility with the set member and avoids premature acceptance of potentially '*wrong*' perceptions.

It is also worthwhile always remembering that the perceptions of any set member giving feedback is their reality (if not our own) and that all set members are shaped by their own mind-sets in terms of how they see the world, the set and the people in it.

> It is folly to say you know what is happening to other people. Only they know. They have their own universes of their own eyes and ears.
>
> *(Douglas Adams)*

Receiving feedback can also be challenging. Good rules of thumb are:

- ***Listen to the feedback before responding***: A kneejerk reaction might well be to respond immediately. Some feedback can certainly be uncomfortable to hear, but ultimately can be beneficial, as it may offer the set member insights which otherwise might be missed.

- ***Be clear about what is being said:*** The set member receiving feedback can check out that what they have heard is accurate before responding to it. They might also wish to hear from other set members and also to get their feedback before responding.
- ***Decide on what action to take:*** When a set member receives feedback they can decide on how valuable it is and the possible consequences of either, on the one hand, ignoring it, or on the other, accepting and deciding to use it as a basis for changed future actions. The choice is entirely that of the set member.

REFLECTION

Action learning adds structure to personal experience by giving time and space for reflection. Reflection on previous actions makes the vital difference between having 10 years' worth of experience or having one year's worth of experience simply repeated nine times. Reflection within sets enables a higher level of awareness of the complexities of the internal ('*in-here*') and the external ('*out-there*') worlds and their inter-connectedness and this is achieved through the support and challenge from set members. Time dedicated to reflection in action learning sets nudges individual set members towards action in the workplace, in part due to the peer pressure from other set members.

As the set gets going, the facilitator role, and that of the set members, tends to move from energising and speeding things up more towards reflecting and slowing things down. This might involve not only possibly asking set members to work together in pairs and reviewing achievements to date, but also encouraging set members to take responsibility for their actions; seeing themselves as (at least partly) the cause of what happens to them; not blaming themselves for these actions and finally, to enhance their learning by generalising from their experience.

> Everything looks like a failure in the middle.
>
> *(Rosabeth Moss Kanter)*

LEARNING TO COPE WITHOUT A 'TEACHER' OR A 'TRAINER'

For many set members, being a member of an action learning set can feel like a strange experience. Their typical experience will be sitting in a '*classroom*' setting with other learners and a '*teacher*', '*lecturer*' or a '*trainer*'. In an action learning set some of these features are repeated – but the teacher or trainer does not teach them anything! This problem can be addressed by acknowledging the likely feelings of discomfort which set members may experience; by structuring the equal time-sharing for set members; by the facilitator emphasising a willingness to co-operatively support the overall learning process, and by encouraging the taking of first steps by set members. If, for example, the set members are only writing down notes from what the facilitator is saying, the facilitator will certainly need to point this out to them!

LINKING LEARNING WITH WORK

For many people joining an action learning set the world of work and the world of learning are not at all linked. The former is seen as the arena of acting and doing, whereas the latter is concerned with reflecting and conceptualising (4). The choice of the issue or project by the set members and their sponsors within their organisations can help to link these two, seemingly distinct, spheres. If the issue chosen is too much like ordinary work, then it may not be seen by the set member as a source of rich learning. If it is too untypical of ordinary work, then it may not be seen as relevant, although that will depend on the ability of the set member to conceptualise the linkages between work and learning. The facilitator and the other set members have a key role to play here, but other things which can help include ensuring that the issues chosen have an inter-professional, inter-departmental or inter-organisational focus; ensuring that frontline staff have to interact with senior managers in order to pursue their topic, and by requiring contact in order to address the topic with patients, clients, service users, carers and other potential stakeholders.

> The future of work consists of learning a living.
>
> *(Marshall McLuhan)*

LEARNING FROM COLLEAGUES

While Revans called set members '*comrades in adversity*', a number of other things can also help the process of learning from colleagues. One is the notion of needs and offers. At the beginning of an action learning programme (and potentially at intervals during the programme) there can be real value in the facilitator asking set members to write down what they want and what they have to offer – and then posting the results on a flipchart for all set members to see. This process can lead to person-to-person linkages of the kind '*I see you need to know more about compassionate care. I attended a workshop on this a couple of months ago and applied it with my staff – and I'd be happy to talk it through with you.*' However, it can take some time for this process to get going, as people can feel '*selfish*' in addressing their own hopes and fears, and may believe that this personal and local action cannot possibly be enriching and illuminating for their fellow set members.

BEING A TEMPERED RADICAL

While individuals who become members of an action learning set usually identify with, and are committed to, their own employing organisations, the insights which typically come from such involvement can also commit them to a set of core values or a cause which may differ fundamentally from the dominant culture of their organisations. They are positioned on the boundary – both inside and outside their organisations – as a basis for their judgements and actions. As such they are '*tempered radicals*', that is:

> People who want to succeed in their organisations, yet want to live by their values or identities, even if they are somehow at odds with the dominant culture of their organisations.

They want to fit in organisationally, but they also want to retain what it is that makes them different – to rock the boat, but also to stay in it. This is an ambivalent position and requires a careful balancing act on the part of the individual in deciding, for example, what course of action to pursue, how far to push and when to hold back (5,6). The dangers which tempered radicals have to guard against include:

- A possible sense of despair at the implications of adopting a radical analysis of their professional or organisational context
- A developing feeling of '*lost innocence*' as they question their own taken-for-granted assumptions
- A growing feeling of '*impostership*' as they doubt their own worthiness to question their organisation or their profession
- Experiencing a feeling of '*cultural suicide*' as they then encounter the disbelief and possible hostility of colleagues when they question or challenge accepted professional and organisational practices (7)

The fellowship and support of the other set members enable such tempered radicals to work through the dangers and risks that inevitably come from working on difficult problems.

REFERENCES

1. G. Egan, *The Skilled Helper: A Problem-Management Approach to Helping* (Belmont, CA: Brooks-Cole Publishing, 1993).
2. C. Argyris, *Knowledge for Action: A Guide to Overcoming Barriers to Organisational Change* (San Francisco, CA: Jossey-Bass, 1993).
3. J. Edmonstone, *Personal Resilience for Healthcare Staff: When the Going Gets Tough* (London: Radcliffe Publishing, 2013).
4. D. Kolb, *Experiential Learning* (Englewood Cliffs, NJ: Prentice-Hall, 1984).
5. D. Myerson and M. Scully, Tempered radicals and the politics of radicalism and change, *Organisation Science* 6 (5); 1995: 585–600.
6. D. Myerson, *Tempered Radicals: How Everyday Leaders Inspire Change at Work* (Boston: Harvard Business School Press, 2003).
7. S. Brookfield, Tales from the darkside: A phenomenology of adult critical reflection, *International Journal of Lifelong Education* 13 (3): 203–216.

9

Supporting, recording, ending

SUPPORTING ACTION LEARNING THROUGH DIAGNOSTICS

> The real voyage of discovery consists not in seeking new lands, but with seeing with new eyes.
>
> *(Marcel Proust)*

There exists a wide range of support material and activities that can be used as part of the action learning process. Some of these are contained in Part 3 of this book. All this material, however, should be used with great care and discrimination, for there is a danger of confusing means with ends – a case of the tail wagging the dog. Nevertheless, such support material may be helpful because of the innate and overwhelming seductiveness of the issue being addressed by the set member, which may lead them to become completely obsessed with action, at the expense of learning. Support material can therefore be useful in diverting people away from such task obsession and towards learning about the processes by which the task is achieved. Good support material forces explicit discussion within the set of the learning processes and achievements within the workplace ('*out there*') and within the set ('*in here*'). Support material should really only be used when:

- It has been presented and described to the set members by the facilitator.
- Set members have had sufficient time and opportunity to consider the advantages and disadvantages of using such material.
- Individual set members and the set as a whole make a conscious decision to use the material.

A number of questionnaire-based diagnostics exist which can help set members to assess their own personal styles and preferences. These include, for example, the Myers-Briggs Type Inventory (MBTI) and the Thomas-Kilman Conflict Mode Instrument. However, the most relevant diagnostics may be those that focus on individual learning styles. The original work in this field was undertaken by David Kolb (1) and his ideas, especially on learning and problem solving, are clearly reflected in action learning, although they do embody an essentially rationalistic approach. The self-diagnostic method which he created – the Learning Style Inventory (LSI) – has, however, often been criticised for being highly culture bound and has found less favour as time has passed. The Learning Styles Questionnaire (LSQ) devised by Peter Honey and Alan Mumford (2) has proved much more popular. It identifies four learning styles:

- ***Activist*:** Someone who likes to take direct action and who thrives on learning from challenges and from new experiences. Activists are enthusiastic and welcome new challenges and experiences, but are less interested in what has happened in the past or in putting things into a broader context. They are primarily interested in the here and now. They like to have a go, to try things out and to participate.
- ***Reflector*:** Someone who likes to think about things in detail before taking action, so they tend to be cautious, standing back and observing experiences from different perspectives. They take a thoughtful approach, are good listeners and prefer to adopt a low profile.
- ***Theorist*:** Someone who likes to see how things fit into an overall pattern. They are logical and objective '*systems*' people who prefer a sequential approach to problems. They are analytical, pay great attention to detail and adapt and integrate their observations into logically sound theories.
- ***Pragmatist*:** Someone who likes to see how things work out in practice. They are practical, down-to-earth and like to solve problems, trying out new ideas, theories and techniques to see whether they actually work in practice.

While everyone develops their own characteristic profile across these four styles, a person's learning style is not something which is fixed and is certainly capable of change, particularly in response to a variety of different external situations and influences, such as a change of work setting. Moreover, the information which is derived from the LSQ results should never be used to avoid particular types of learning, but should provide a basis for developing an approach to personal learning which reflects a more balanced profile.

An action learning set is most valuable to individuals when different learning styles are represented within the set membership, and least useful where the individual set members all have the same or similar learning styles. People with different learning style preferences, often derived from different areas of experience, typically make the best set members precisely because their line of thought provokes the most challenging and enlightening questions from each other.

There is an obvious danger, however, of using the LSQ as a typology – as a means of dividing people into discreet categories. When people pin labels on themselves (such as '*I'm a Pragmatist*') they might possibly believe that, once they have identified their predominant learning style, it is a fixed and predominant personality trait which cannot be changed, so they must always work within that particular limitation, seeking only those experiences which match their preferred style – and hence avoid those that offer a potentially different approach. Such a viewpoint runs counter to the understandings about adult learning outlined in Chapter 1. Used with care and sensitivity, the LSQ can support action learning – but with the rider that it must never be mistaken for an end in itself, as its' only practical use is as a means to help and to stimulate the learning process.

SUPPORTING ACTION LEARNING THROUGH LEARNING DIARIES

The purpose of a learning diary is twofold: firstly, to record the set member's experience across the duration of the set meetings, and secondly to make linkages between what happens in the set and what happens in the workplace, in order to encourage and to develop reflection on experience. If a learning diary is adopted by an individual set member then they will need to be completely frank and sincere in what they write and will need to exercise a real degree of self-discipline in order to find the time and space to update the learning diary on a regular basis. This reflective process can be aided by including, for example, relevant cartoons, newspaper or journal clippings, quotable quotes and so on.

To encourage learning, a diary will need to be both sequential and reflective.

- ***Sequential***: This involves jotting down notes on a continuing and regular basis under such headings as:
    - ***People***: The behaviour of people in the work situation or in the set who make an important impact on the set member
    - ***Events***: Key incidents that take place at work or in the set meeting
    - ***Reactions:*** What the set member thought, felt, wanted and did
- ***Reflective***: This involves consideration of:
    - ***Insights***: Ideas or thoughts that made a significant impact on the set member – either their own contributions or alternatively those of other set members
    - ***Learning***: The sense that the set member makes of what's happening to themselves and others

Reflective learning can be stimulated by such questions as:

'When did I feel most engaged?' 'And why?'
'When did I feel most distanced?' 'And why?'
'When did I feel most puzzled?' 'And why?'
'When did I feel most affirmed?' 'And why?'
'What gaps in my learning did I discover and how should I go about filling them?'

In this way, a learning diary seeks to be both **retrospective** (looking back and aiming to understand what has happened) and **prospective** (looking forward and aiming to decide what to do next).

RECORDING

What happens in an action learning set meeting is certainly not what happens in a formal and structured meeting where the minutes capture the issues that were covered, the discussion that took place and the decisions that were made, but there can be real value in keeping a record of what goes on in the set meeting. This can take the form of notes, mind maps, pictures, symbols or metaphors or quotations which capture an important learning point. There can thus be merit in asking, at each set meeting, for one person to be responsible for taking brief notes and then copying and circulating these, especially for agreed actions or requests for specific resources or information. Figure 9.1 offers one template for recording what goes on in a set meeting.

Individual set members will also want to record what the set meeting meant to them and the **Set Meeting Review Worksheet** in Part 3 of this book provides a useful means of doing so.

Date of meeting	
Venue	
Present	
Apologies	
Issues discussed	
Outcomes	
Matters to follow-up	
What?	
How?	
By whom?	
By when?	
Date of next meeting	
Venue of next meeting	
Time of next meeting	

Figure 9.1 Recording what goes on in a set meeting.

ENDING

Although almost all action learning sets are created for an agreed and finite time period, there is often a strong desire on the part of the set members for the life of the set to continue after it is '*officially*' over. This may be because, for some set members, the combination of support and challenge which they receive from colleagues in the set is fairly unique in relation to the remainder of their work or life experience. Yet action learning sets are not permanent entities, so the issue of the '*shelf life*' of sets is important.

Given the level of commitment that is required from set members, every set will need to review regularly whether it is continuing to meet the individual needs of set members and there will inevitably come a time when that particular configuration of people and issues is no longer effective. Sets which continue to meet, either out of habit, or because it is comfortable to do so, will not really be productive, and this will soon become obvious.

Ending the life of a set should never be seen as a failure. Instead it is a good test of action learning itself if the set knows when it is right to stop, rather than continuing on in a sterile manner. If the set has been working well then it should be mature enough to realise that as much has been achieved as can be achieved and that the time has come to stop. The ending of the set is therefore part of the development process itself and a symbol of growth, rather than of loss.

The final session of a set might well include the following activities:

- Set members personally recapturing the way they felt when first coming to the set.
- Reflecting on the original aims and outcomes of the set, and so discovering what each set member has achieved since the set commenced, and hence providing a reminder of how far each set member has come.
- Reflecting on the experience of being in the set by remembering how it had been along the way.
- Set members sharing with each other how they are now feeling at the end of the set's life, and saying their personal and group goodbyes before moving on.

Some set members part in a flood of emotion, others simply slip away and others will wish to celebrate in some fashion or another. Some sets may continue to meet, but socially rather than for the former purposes. Others may continue as virtual sets, communicating by other means.

The processes which set members have gone through and the relationships which they have built, fostered and maintained will prove valuable to them even after the set has ended, and in a variety of settings. The lessons learned by set members will therefore continue to resonate long after the set has gone.

REFERENCES

1. D. Kolb, *Experiential Learning* (Englewood Cliffs, NJ: Prentice-Hall, 1984).
2. P. Honey and A. Mumford, *Using Your Learning Styles*, Second edition (Maidenhead: Peter Honey Publications, 1995).

10

Dealing with anxiety in action learning

> The range of what we think and do is limited by what we fail to notice, and because we fail to notice that we fail to notice, there is little we can do to change, until we notice how failing to notice shapes our thoughts and deeds.
>
> *(Ronald Laing)*

The success of action learning sets can potentially be put at risk by both non-activity and by activity, such as:

NON-ACTIVITY

- Not having a real-time and relevant issue to bring to the set meetings
- Set members not attending set meetings or not following through on the commitments to action which they had previously given at those meetings
- Not preparing for set meetings – simply turning-up and expecting '*something*' to happen, with the onus for making it happen being on the other set members and/or the facilitator
- Passive attendance, or being there in body but not in mind. Not listening or responding to what is being said by others

ACTIVITY

- Yarn-spinning and using up of time
- Theorising – shifting the focus from the issue itself towards theories and concepts about the issue
- Game-playing and undermining others' serious commitment
- Hogging the spotlight and dominating the agenda
- Gossiping – wasting time and avoiding addressing the real issues

Why does this happen? What takes place in an action learning set is not solely a rational or an intellectual process. Every individual set member will have, in the past, experienced both positive and negative learning experiences which they view inevitably through the template of their own emotional and psychological history. Such experiences will also have been shaped and conditioned through membership of family, work, professional, organisational and social groupings and have been conditioned by broader economic, social and political forces operating in both work organisations and in the wider society.

Because effective action learning involves risk (of failure, but also of success), it also always involves anxiety. Anxiety is an integral part of being a set member (and also a set facilitator) and can contribute to both the success and failure of sets. Since action learning is open-ended, unpredictable and emergent, anxiety is probably endemic. The contrast is with more conventional training approaches where the uncertainty is constrained and order seemingly established through educational curricula, adherence to best practices and reliance on set techniques (1). Anxiety often therefore gets in the way of set members experimenting with new behaviour. Typical examples of anxiety-induced behaviour include:

- ***A reluctance to join in***: An unwillingness to be playful and creative with behaviour and ideas. A reluctance to ask '*What if ... ?*' questions, resulting in highly '*serious*' behaviour.
- ***A narrow self-view***: A low self-assessment of personal abilities and resources with a resulting '*resource myopia*' – an inability or unwillingness to recognise the contribution that might be made to helping other set members to address their issues.
- ***Fear of losing face***: Of being perceived as having admitted incompetence or having backed down.
- ***Fear of recrimination***: Because other people (set members or colleagues in the workplace) might misunderstand a set member's changed behaviour and so get angry and resentful.
- ***Fear of losing control***: And ending up in a bigger mess than the current one.
- ***Fear of failure***: In the eyes of other set members, the facilitator (perhaps perceived as being an '*authority*' figure) and of other colleagues in the work organisation. People who fear the possibility of failure will experience difficulty in taking even calculated risks, will undervalue the importance of feelings and will seldom be spontaneous in their interactions with others.
- ***Fear of ambiguity***: An avoidance of matters which lack clarity or where outcomes are unknown or unpredictable. A reluctance to try something out, to see whether it works or not, and an overemphasis on the known at the expense of the unknown.
- ***Fear of disorder***: A dislike of complexity (usually labelled as '*confusion*') and a preference for order, structure and balance, often expressed in terms of opposites, such as good versus bad and right versus wrong, with a corresponding failure to appreciate and integrate the best from these seemingly polarised viewpoints.
- ***Fear of looking foolish***: And attracting negative comments about having acted out of character.
- ***Fear of being vulnerable***: Of not really knowing what will happen as a result of trying a different approach.
- ***Fear of letting someone else make a big mistake***: When feeling responsible for what the other person does.
- ***Fear of influencing others***: A concern not to appear as aggressive or '*pushy*' and thus a hesitation in identifying with emerging points of view.

The sources of such anxiety may include the set member's own work role and the local setting in which it operates; the particular nature of the issue that they are working on; uncertainty over the purpose and nature of the set itself and of the set member's place within it. All professional staff working in statutory and voluntary agencies, particularly those delivering human services (2), also suffer from anxiety because of the discretionary nature of much of their work (3,4).

> In order to arrive at what you do not know you must go by the way that is the way of ignorance.
>
> *(T.S. Eliot)*

Such in-built immunities to change often lead to avoidance behaviour or to '*defensive routines*' (5) – unconscious strategies for self-protection, which unfortunately inhibit the potential to learn and to become more effective. These defensive thoughts and feelings have been acquired over time and through experience because it is believed that they keep us safe, but incongruously, they are very often the source of our failure – the very reason that we remain stuck in behaviour patterns that result in repeated error.

Anxiety can have destructive or self-limiting effects, but can also potentially provide the energy which is needed in order to risk being honest, direct, challenging and different – and so can help to shape and to inform set members' authority and involvement in set meetings, in addition to the self-insight which is also generated. Confronting anxiety may require set members to relinquish their earlier roles, ideas and practices; to create, find or discover new and more adaptable ideas, ways of thinking and acting, and to cope with the instability of changing conditions and the insecurity which change always provokes.

One way of dealing with anxiety is the tendency, especially in work settings, to seek sanctuary in the views of experts. Such people seem to provide anxiety-reducing answers and so offer what can seem like safety and security. By contrast, action learning concentrates on helping people to own and focus on *their* problem – with all the messiness, confusion and uncertainty which that entails – rather than relying upon such expert advice. It encourages people to balance and to optimise the paradoxes facing them in groups and organisations, to experiment and develop their own solutions, rather than appropriating someone else's, and it emphasises the set member learning how to learn, through the use of the set as a facilitating structure or holding framework, where people can express their worries, hopes and fears. It provides the necessary time and space that people need in order to reflect, review, develop understanding and plan ahead. The minimal structure provided by the set, chiefly through the establishment of agreed ground rules, provides a means of containing set members' anxiety, as shown in Figure 10.1.

In the operation of action learning sets it is also sometime possible to observe the phenomenon of '*parallel processing*' – dysfunctional behaviour which is reported as being manifest in a workplace setting also being visible in the working of the set. Where this does exist then there is an onus on the set members and the facilitator to identify and name the (in-set) behaviour, linking it to the reported organisational context and encouraging the set member concerned to address it.

This issue of anxiety seems particularly true within '*human service organisations*' (2), such as health, social and community care, the police, the clergy and so on, where a major part of the work of professional staff is '*emotional labour*', defined as:

> The suppression of feeling in order to sustain an outward appearance that produces in others a sense of being cared for. (6)

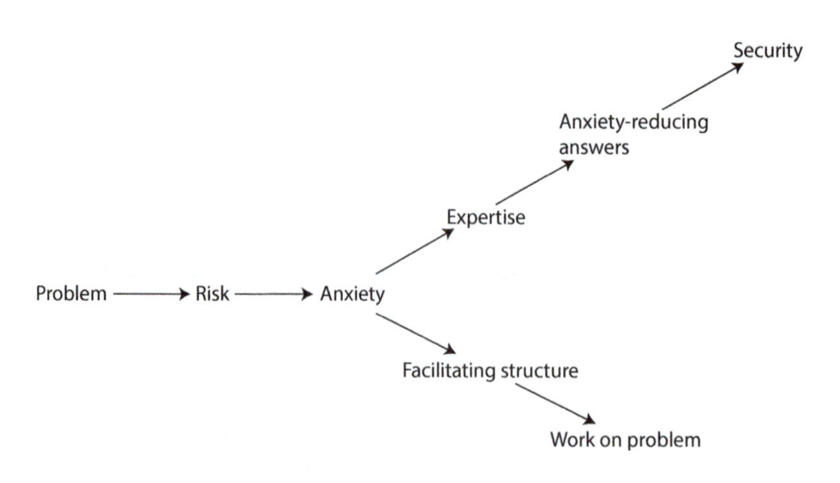

Figure 10.1 Alternative means of dealing with anxiety.

While this is true of the practice of individual professionals, there is also an organisational impact. In healthcare it has been suggested that:

> Organisations operate in society as 'containers' of the emotions and anxieties of patients' relatives and families and because of this the experience of leaders and managers of clinical professional staff is different from that of an industrial or commercial enterprise. Managerial initiatives from the 1980s onwards have served to increase and bolster the potential defence mechanisms in play to deal with the inherent anxiety of working in healthcare. Increased bureaucratisation of professional work has also served to increase prescription and decrease discretion. (7)

The value of the action learning set is that it provides a holding and enabling framework – a transitional space – in which set members' sometimes powerful and frightening anxieties can be faced, comprehended and worked – although with the appropriate balance of support and challenge from the other set members and the facilitator. They can help to build the confidence of what Revans called their '*comrades in adversity*' through empathising with each set member's emotional state at the time that they are describing their issue; by seeking to enhance increasing levels of respect and trust within the set; by modelling appropriate behaviour to each other, and by addressing such matters directly, rather than indirectly and implicitly. This helps to build what has been called '*negative capability*', a term originally coined by the poet John Keats, which he described as a state in which a person:

> is capable of being in uncertainties, mysteries, doubts without any irritable reaching after facts and reason. (8)

Such a capability is often the first step on a journey towards greater self-insight, a greater capacity to learn from experience and greater awareness of the political and cultural dimensions of organisational change. It is increasingly needed in present-day organisations, full as they are of contradiction and paradox (9). It takes time to develop, but can be done. Some of the ways include:

- Acknowledging that anxiety is probably likely to be present within the set
- Identifying the differences between action learning and conventional education and training approaches
- Ensuring that sets are set up properly, as outlined in Chapter 5
- Modelling the legitimate and measured expression of anxiety within the set

> Our deepest fear is not that we are inadequate. Our deepest fear is that we are powerful beyond measure. It is our light, not our darkness, that frightens us. We ask ourselves 'Who am I to be brilliant, gorgeous, talented and fabulous?' Actually, who are you not to be? You are a child of God. Your playing small doesn't serve the world. There's nothing enlightened about shrinking so that other people won't feel insecure around you. We were born to make manifest the glory of God that is within us. It's not just in some of us; it's in everyone. And as we let our own light shine, we unconsciously give other people permission to do the same. As we are liberated from our own fear, our presence automatically liberates others.
>
> *(Nelson Mandela)*

REFERENCES

1. M. Pedler and C. Abbott, *Facilitating Action Learning: A Practitioner's Guide* (Maidenhead: Open University Press, 2013).
2. J. Edmonstone, Human service organisations: Implications for management and organisation development, *Management Education and Development* 13 (3); 1982: 163–173.
3. E. Jaques, *A General Theory of Bureaucracy* (London: Heinemann, 1976).
4. J. Dowie and A. Elstein, *Professional Judgement: A Reader in Clinical Decision-Making* (Cambridge: Cambridge University Press, 1988).
5. C. Argyris, *Strategy, Change and Defensive Routines* (London: Pitman Publishing, 1985).
6. R. Hayward and M. Tuckey, Emotions in uniform: How nurses regulate emotions at work via emotional boundaries, *Human Relations* 64 (11); 2011: 1501–1523.
7. J. Edmonstone, What is wrong with NHS leadership development, *British Journal of Healthcare Management* 19 (11); 2013: 8–18.
8. J. Keats, *The Complete Poetical Works and Letters of John Keats* (Cambridge: Houghton Mifflin, 1899).
9. John Edmonstone, Action learning, performativity and negative capability, *Action Learning: Research & Practice* 13 (2); 2016: 139–147.

11

Facilitating action learning sets

> Double vision does not require us to stop and think, but the capacity to keep alive, in the midst of action, a multiplicity of views of a situation.
>
> *(Donald Schon)*

Most action learning sets begin life with a facilitator who is there to enable the learning process to take place by helping to create those conditions which make it possible for set members to learn from their own experience and from that of their colleagues. The facilitator, who can emerge from a wide variety of backgrounds, is not there to lead the set, to chair it or to control it. They are the '*guide on the side*', rather than the '*sage on the stage*'. It is a role more to be learnt than to be taught.

Inevitably, the facilitator is most active in the early life of the set, involved in setting it up, in helping set members to find their feet, getting to know each other, seeking agreement on ground rules and so on. All this is intended to '*jump-start*' the set, without excessive use of Programmed Knowledge. So the facilitator's intentions need to be limited to where and when real help can be given; so they need to be judicious – wise and careful; and to be tentative – and therefore gentle and timely. All this is based on the overriding intention of being helpful and fostering learning.

As the set gets going, the facilitator role, and that of the set members, tends to move from that of energising and speeding things up towards one of slowing things down and encouraging reflection much more. This can involve not only asking the set members to work together, perhaps in pairs, and reviewing their own and the set's achievements to date, but also in encouraging set members to take responsibility for their actions; to seeing themselves as potentially the cause of what happens to them; not blaming themselves for these actions and finally, to enhancing their learning by generalising from their experience.

Energy levels in action learning sets can vary. Sometimes set members can feel '*fired-up*' and involved, but on other occasions they can '*wilt*' and a sense of hopelessness can sometimes develop. The set facilitator should therefore be sensitive to these mood changes but should always simply reflect on what they see, rather than trying to '*lift*' the set. There are, however, some things which can help to develop a sense of stamina for the set, and these include:

- Sharing both telephone numbers and email addresses so that set members can be in contact with each other between set meetings, can check-out each other's progress and can offer encouragement to one another.
- Encouraging set members to meet in pairs and trios between the dates of agreed set meetings.

- Setting-up helping pairs where each set member keeps the other in mind and makes contact with them regularly.
- Arranging an informal lunchtime meeting, halfway between regular set meetings.
- Encouraging set members to identify two or three actions that they can take before the next meeting.

It will also be important for the facilitator to ask the set members for their suggestions when such a dip occurs, as this will develop their sense of ownership and will encourage further creative ideas.

So the qualities required by facilitators (1) include:

- **Tolerance of ambiguity:** The facilitator constantly operates in a realm of uncertainty and therefore must be prepared to let the set members take control. Unless the facilitator accepts and welcomes this, they will not undertake the facilitator role well and will certainly not enjoy it.
- **Openness and frankness:** An ability to recognise and to express their personal feelings as they arise in the course of a set meeting.
- **Patience:** In endless quantities, as the set members will work within the set and back in the workplace at different speeds.
- **An overwhelming desire to see people learn:** The learning of set members is likely to happen slowly, incrementally, personally and often privately. So powerful can be the desire to speed things up that the facilitator will inevitably spend some of their time '*biting their tongue*' and not intervening for fear of upsetting the learning process in the set, for both individuals and for the set as a whole. A good facilitator will also be actively encouraging the involvement of all set members, particularly those who may be quiet or who seem withdrawn.
- **Empathy:** A sense of standing in another's shoes and seeing the world through their eyes.
- **Self-doubt:** The ability to question oneself, to admit to personal uncertainties and mistakes in a way that does not in any way threaten the security of the set, but instead reveals that the facilitator is human too. The facilitator thus demonstrates self-insight by being open and frank about their own feelings, but not to the extent of letting these feelings dominate the proceedings and so threaten the security of the set.
- **Proportion:** An ability to both summarise and to see the '*big picture*', pulling all the strands together to make sense of what is happening, combined with an awareness of the broader context within which the life and work of the set and its members takes place.
- **Micro-politics:** A skilled facilitator will make it his or her business to understand the micro-politics of the organisation or organisations that they are concerned with – with how things get done, with where the power lies and how it might be mobilised.
- **Role-model:** The facilitator needs to constantly model the behaviour that s/he espouses – to '*walk the talk*' so that there is a match between what they say and what they do.

Some would also claim that a track record of experience in the profession or field concerned can be helpful, although the danger might be that this could be seductive and could potentially lead the facilitator into adopting an expert role (2).

The skills which the action learner then does need to develop include:

- **Skills in asking good questions:** Questions which make set members to both think and feel, but simultaneously to feel both supported and challenged, rather than criticised.

- **Skills in choosing issues that help:** Out of everything that might be going on at any one time within the set, the facilitator needs to track and choose those matters that link what is happening in the set with the parallel difficulties reported by set members back in their work organisations.
- **Skills in using the right language:** Different professional and occupational tribes have different '*languages*' made up of jargon and abbreviations. The rule for the facilitator, however, has always to be '*only connect*', so they need to be highly aware of the dangers of potential mystification, talking-down or the seduction of intellectualising.
- **The skill of being truthfully helpful:** Making statements truthfully, while structuring such statements to be of maximum benefit to both individual set members or to the whole set.
- **Skills in the timing of interventions:** Too early and the issue can fail to be understood; too late and the opportunity for learning may be lost.
- **The skill of saying nothing and being invisible:** Realising that sometimes to intervene at crucial points may interrupt or short-circuit an individual set member's learning process, or that of the set as a whole.
- **Skills in calibrating action and learning:** If the bulk of the set members' talk is about what they have learned, then the facilitator may need to ask '*But what are you going to do?*'. Similarly, if the majority of the talk is about action, then the facilitator may need to enquire '*So what exactly is this saying to you?*'

What are not needed are the following, which can impede the learning of set members:

- **Trainer skills:** As the content of set meetings is brought by the set members, there is no need to formally structure the sequencing of sessions, to prepare material and to adopt an expert role.
- **Presentation skills:** The more effective the facilitator is with these skills, the more likely it will be that set members will see them as an expert; the more passive they are likely to be and the less likely as a result that they will be to take responsibility for their own development.
- **Fluency:** The use of language in an oratorical sense detracts from the facilitator's need to express exactly what they see and feel in an authentic manner.

So what are the desirable characteristics, experience, competence and track record that a facilitator might need?

- A first requirement would simply be that the facilitator had certainly experienced **being an action learning set member** before taking on the facilitator role.
- The facilitator should also have had experience of **facilitating a number of different action learning sets** – the wider the variety, then the more comprehensive the experience.
- The facilitator should be capable of drawing, wherever appropriate, on useful **theoretical models** to illustrate what may be happening in the set or back in the workplace. Insights drawn from other fields, such as literature, poetry and so on, can also be useful.
- The facilitator should have **working experience of a wide range of helpful tools**, both for use in the set meetings and to assist set members on their return to the workplace. A compendium of these is offered in Part 3 of this book.
- The facilitator should be able to **give evidence of some kind of supervisory relationship** – this might be on a one-to-one basis or on a group basis (such as membership of a facilitated set of action learning facilitators).

- The facilitator should be able to produce **a portfolio of both formal and informal evidence** supporting the above. This might include, for example, evaluation reports, journal articles and testimonials from set members, sponsors, champions and other stakeholders.

FACILITATOR DEVELOPMENT

There are three major routes for the development of facilitators:

- ***Self-development*:** This involves the individual development of facilitator practice, not conducted through any formally taught programme, but by way of observation, co-facilitation, mentoring by an experienced facilitator, coaching, reflective practice, reading, writing and so on. There is no validation at all by any external body. This is the route by which many people start, particularly those who have already had the valuable experience of being a set member, and such a route can be very successful, especially if the individual concerned has access to support.
- ***Proprietary or private training*:** This is typically delivered through a taught programme based upon a specific in-house model or approach to action learning. Such programmes are usually focused on the more practical aspects of facilitation and the particular methods of practice approved by the programme deliverer or client organisation. This route may lead to an in-house award, recognised by the awarding organisation. Examples of this would include the World Institute of Action Learning (WIAL). Alternatively, such programmes may be quality-assured against the provider's own curriculum, such as a development programme by the UK's Institute of Leadership and Management (ILM). Logs of practice or mini case studies are typically used as evidence for satisfactory attendance and completion of the programme. This route is somewhat problematic in terms of quality control, as, given the range of particular preferences for models and approaches, it can be difficult to identify exactly which approach to action learning is being offered.
- ***Qualification recognised by a regulatory body; usually a taught programme, against a recognised framework or standard*:** This route generally takes a broader approach to understanding the different perspectives on, and variants of, action learning, coupled with critical reflection of the facilitator's own practice, together with guided study of the underpinning concepts and theory. This approach leads to formally assessed and accredited qualifications, such as the standards for action learning facilitators regulated by the UK's Office of Qualifications and Examinations Regulation (OFQUAL) and as offered by the ILM. Also falling within this route are university-accredited programmes that map on to the standards set by the UK's Higher Education Academy.

Even if the latter two routes are followed, the necessity for self-development by the facilitator remains a constant factor, not least because personal commitment and personal example are perceived by set members as being vital. The desire to work as a facilitator of action learning (based significantly on an adherence to the ethos of action learning) and the skills and knowledge that are acquired are part of a complete '*package*'. Continuing self-development as a facilitator can be by a range of different means, including:

- ***A facilitators set*:** The creation of a '*meta-set*' comprising facilitators alone, whose challenges relate to the work of facilitating other sets, can be a powerful means of continuing development, as well as providing a means of professional supervision for facilitators (3).

- ***Reading***: There are a number of useful introductions to action learning, some generic in nature and others relating to health, social and community care. The best of these are:
  - Mike Pedler and Christine Abbott: *Facilitating Action Learning: A Practitioners Guide* (Maidenhead: Open University Press, 2013)
  - John Edmonstone: *Action Learning In Healthcare: A Practical Handbook* (London: Radcliffe Publishing, 2011)
  - Christine Abbott and Paul Taylor: *Action Learning In Social Work* (London: Sage, 2013)

  In addition, the journal *Action Learning: Research & Practice* is published three times a year by Taylor & Francis Group (www.tandfonline.com/toc/CALR20/current#.VM9iEGisWT8).
- ***Writing***: Keeping a personal journal based on the experience of working with action learning can be a valuable aid to self-reflection on practice. Turning such material into an '*account of practice*' in order to share with a wider audience of action learning set members and facilitators means making it accessible and relevant to such a wider community. The journal *Action Learning: Research & Practice* always welcomes such contributions.

PITFALLS FOR FACILITATORS

Although action learning provides a great opportunity for lively and engaged learning, there can also be pitfalls which facilitators need to be aware of. Some of these relate to the operation of the set, while others relate to the facilitator's behaviour.

Set-based pitfalls

The most common pitfall is for the focus on action and learning to be lost. As a meeting of like minds, an obvious function of the set is a social one – meeting with colleagues to share highs and lows, achievements and anxieties and to generally '*touch base*'. While there is real value in all of these things, it is important not to lose sight of the full range of learning opportunities offered by the set. So some of the dangers include:

- ***Some set members may have been 'volunteered'or even 'sent'***: Such individuals have not themselves decided to be part of a set and so believe, consciously or unconsciously, that they have been sent for remedial purposes – to '*sort them out*'. The facilitator, if aware of such background, might discuss this personally with the set member themselves, and with their sponsor, seeking to ascertain whether set membership is appropriate for them or not.
- ***There is a lack of organisational support***: If membership of the set is perceived in the set member's organisation as a '*waste of time*' or a '*jolly holiday*', then this could seriously affect the credibility of the outcomes of a set meeting and the consistency of attendance. Adequate preparation should avoid this, but it may sometimes be necessary for the facilitator to explain matters clearly to the set member's sponsor.
- ***Some set members don't pull their weight and leave it to others to do all the work***: Such a problem needs to be dealt with earlier, rather than later because the longer it is left, the more damage will be done to the set and so its members are likely to become resentful. The issue may need to be placed on the agenda of a set meeting and to be addressed directly, based on how the set members feel about it. Such a discussion needs to be conducted in positive terms, asking, for example, what can be done to ensure that everyone has the chance to contribute.

- ***There seems to be a lack of time*:** It is far better to work effectively on a couple of set members' issues than to cram everyone in to a limited time. Time spent at the beginning of a set meeting agreeing on the use of time is therefore time well spent.
- ***The set spends too much time working out what people should be doing, rather than discussing issues and learning from each other's experiences*:** This can be tackled early by devoting time at the first meeting of the set so that everyone understands the requisite way of working.
- ***Set members wander off the point during set meetings and generally have trouble staying focused*:** One way of dealing with this can be to have a written agenda or timetable for each set meeting. The facilitator can also check with set members whether they consider that set meetings are going on too long. Enthusiasm and concentration cannot be maintained indefinitely but can be refreshed and maximised by short and frequent breaks, such as coffee, tea and lunch breaks, by '*comfort stops*' and by regular changes of tack.

Facilitator's behaviour pitfalls

Such pitfalls typically derive from the facilitator mistaking their own needs for those of the set members. An obvious example would be the tendency for set members to leave it to the facilitator only to notice what is going on in the set and to ask questions, rather than set members taking on that responsibility themselves. Other pitfalls include:

- ***The temptation of the expert role*:** The danger that, by falling back on the expert role, the facilitator encourages passivity among set members – and so promotes a corresponding false sense of confidence in the facilitator!
- ***The seduction of rescuing*:** This can happen when a facilitator gives in to the urge to rescue a set member who is struggling with a particularly difficult question, and offers them specific suggestions about what they must do to resolve their issue.
- ***Mistaking the means as the end*:** This involves '*padding out*' the work of the set with small and incremental assignments which, over time, change the process of the set meeting into that of a more traditional learning programme. The caveats mentioned in Chapter 9 about the use of support material apply especially here.

DEALING WITH DIFFICULT SET MEMBERS

From time to time a facilitator will encounter a set member whose behaviour is disruptive of the learning and action of other set members. This may often come in the form of inappropriate interventions and the following are possible questions which the facilitator might pose. Increasingly, as the set grows in experience, it would be the other set members who would assist and confront each other on such matters.

Can we please stop for a moment and review exactly what's happening here? Bill, can you confirm whose airtime it is?

Betty, that's an important point, but it also sounds like a leading question. Can you please turn it into an open question?

Andy, how do you think you might be sabotaging yourself in working in this set?

Jean, do you realise how you are operating in the set?
Tom, how aware are you about what it's like to be Eric?
Clare, I think that Yvonne might need to finish her line of questioning before you make your contribution. Is that right Yvonne?

A FACILITATOR'S CHECKLIST

What are the things that a facilitator would need to consider when asked to facilitate an action learning set? The following are some key issues which would need to be addressed:

- ***Identify who is the client or clients for the action learning work*:** Who are the major stakeholders and what exactly are their expectations?
- ***Identify exactly what variant of action learning is being called for*:** This may involve having to discuss the variants with the client or clients.
- ***Identify the intended outcomes of the action learning programme*:** How clear is it exactly what it is expected that action learning will achieve? How realistic is this?
- ***Consider the extent to which there is a match between the organisational culture or cultures and the underlying assumptions of action learning*:** If there is a mismatch, should action learning even be being considered?
- ***Consider whether action learning is seen as a strategic or an operational intervention*:** Is the intention to focus solely on small-scale operational concerns or can bigger and more strategic concerns also be addressed?
- ***Identify whether set members are likely to address tame or wicked issues*:** Or more likely what is to be the balance between these two?
- ***Identify who is the organisational champion or champions for action learning*:** If one or several do not exist then the facilitator might consider whether action learning should be being adopted. Alternatively, is it possible to identify some individual or a group which is favourable and then to brief them well, or even to mobilise such a group?
- ***Identify what the 'entry' process is for set members*:** To what extent are they (and their sponsors) realistically prepared?
- ***Identify what the 're-entry' process is for set members*:** After the set membership ceases, how do the organisation or organisations concerned intend to capitalise on the learning and development achieved? Do they have a pre-prepared strategy for doing so? If not, do they require assistance in developing one?
- ***Ensure, as far as possible, that the set membership is voluntary and diverse*:** This could involve discussing criteria for set membership with the client or clients.
- ***Identify a suitable venue for set meetings*:** This should be a quiet place, with no interruptions, equipped with comfortable chairs, flipcharts, pads and pens. Tea, coffee and meal arrangements should be agreed.
- ***Agree on the frequency and duration of set meetings.***
- ***Identify exactly what the evaluation process needs to be*:** Consideration of this needs to take place at the outset rather than retrospectively.

> The test of a first-rate intelligence is the ability to hold two opposed ideas in the mind at the same time and still retain the ability to function.
>
> *(F. Scott Fitzgerald)*

REFERENCES

1. D. Casey, David Casey on the role of the set adviser, in *Action Learning in Practice*, Fourth edition, ed. Mike Pedler (Farnham: Gower Publishing, 2011), 55–64.
2. C. Rigg, Action learning in the public service system: Issues, tension and a future agenda, in *Action Learning, Leadership and Organisational Development in Public Services*, eds. Clare Rigg and Sue Richards (Abingdon: Routledge, 2006), 195–206.
3. Geoff Mead, Developing ourselves as police leaders: How can we enquire collaboratively in hierarchical organisations? in *Action Learning, Leadership and Organisational Development in Public Services*, eds. Clare Rigg and Sue Richards (Abingdon: Routledge, 2006), 117–130.

12

Systemic learning: Action learning organisation-wide

It is clear that some organisations successfully develop cultures and sets of working relationships that encourage positive attitudes to new learning – and by contrast others develop cultures which hold back such attitudes. This consideration is based upon two important variables:

- The willingness of senior people in an organisation to promote individual and organisational learning and to make the necessary resources available in order to achieve this.
- The willingness of staff, both individually and in professional and occupational groups, to approach new learning in a positive and welcoming spirit.

Figure 12.1 illustrates how these two dimensions open up a number of possibilities.

In Quadrant A the expectation would be to find evidence of a high commitment among staff to new learning opportunities, plus a willingness to take risks and to be challenged. This is clearly the most fruitful context within which action learning could be initiated. Quadrant B, on the other hand, defines those situations where staff would be most likely to develop a cynical attitude to the few, if any, development opportunities that might be on offer for them. Alternatively, the attitude that might emerge could be one of frustration and anger when people feel denied opportunities for their personal development. People might then feel that

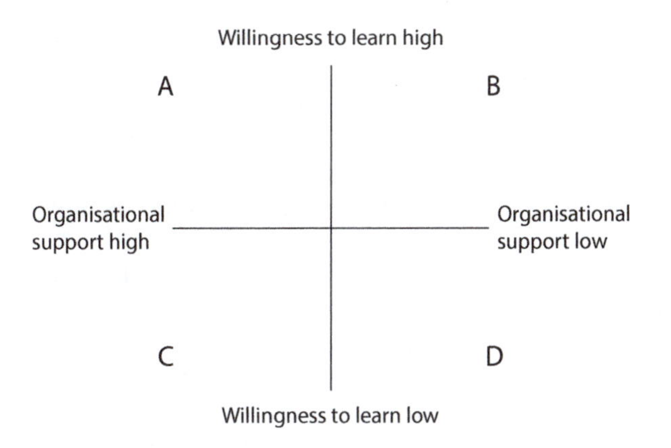

Figure 12.1 Learning and organisational support.

the *'psychological contract'* (1) in relation to their employment is no longer adequate, as they are not offered any real prospect for development through new learning and experience. For organisations that employ well-trained and highly qualified staff this is a serious problem and the evidence suggests that such staff eventually *'vote with their feet'* and leave, taking their knowledge and expertise with them. Many health, social and community care organisations would appear to be of this type.

Quadrant C is where a senior leadership and management team of an organisation is committed to learning, change and development, but their staff appear not to be. Staff continue to rely on their existing skills and knowledge and typically feel major anxiety about the prospect of change. They are uncertain regarding its potential outcomes and so may well be resistant to it, striking a defensive attitude. Quadrant D is an organisational culture in which no new learning seems to take place – a situation where there is no reflection on experience and no real effort to examine or review current practices – a situation described as *'non-learning'* (2). This is often marked by what has been termed *'trained incapacity'*, which has been characterised as:

> ...that state of affairs in which one's abilities function as inadequacies or blind spots. Actions based on training and skills which have been successfully applied in the past may result in inappropriate responses under changed conditions. (3)

Such a state of affairs is also often all too typical of many public service bureaucratic organisations.

It has already been noted that action learning and Organisation Development (OD) are overlapping fields of practice (4). In particular, action learning helps to enhance *'systemic eloquence'* – the ability of parts of a system (an organisation, groups of organisations or a network) to converse well with each other.

Yet there are major barriers or defences which serve to prevent such systemic eloquence, and so hinder organisational learning. These seem to be grounded in an overriding organisational bias for action. Most organisations typically give more value to action and to results than to reflection and inquiry. This activist tendency leads to quick fixes which, in the long-term, may exacerbate the problems faced by organisations if the deeper causes are not addressed. The pressures which reinforce this bias for action include:

- **Time spent in inconclusive deliberations:** One explanation as to why organisations do not learn is that there often seems to be a lack of time, with people feeling too heavily loaded with urgent tasks to engage in any form of reflection. Yet many people also feel frustrated by the amount of time spent in endless, unproductive or unsatisfactory meetings where decisions are not reached or where the same issues permanently reoccur.
- **Urgency of task:** The amount of wasted time spent in such meetings ratchets up the sense of urgency and so, in turn, reduces the willingness to be more reflective. Meetings usually have such tight agendas that there is little or no room left for any in-depth exploration of the issues.
- **Avoidance of reflection, unclear concepts and uncertainty of outcomes:** Deeper reflection may be further avoided because it would mean exposing and experiencing a situation as being much more complex than was originally envisaged, so increasing people's frustration and anxiety. It is not possible to fit the complexities and unpredictability of development practice and organisational life into an idealised and rational model as they are, by their very nature, messy. This can feel highly disturbing, especially for those people who are dominated by a need to always feel in control. Attempts are usually made to minimise

such discomfort by reducing complexity through ever-tighter controls and even more focus on desired outcomes. This then misses opportunities for deeper learning that can actually create greater clarity about the possible choices which might be available. It can also lead to misunderstandings, as there is insufficient space to inquire into the underlying concepts and assumptions.

- **Fear of failure leading to avoidance of decisions:** Uncertainty, anxiety and fear of failure also contribute to large amounts of time being spent in inconclusive meetings and an unproductive '*busyness*'. If a decision feels risky and there is not an environment that supports innovation and learning from mistakes, the result may well be risk-averse behaviour and an avoidance of decisions. Statements such as '*Well, we could do that, except that no-one in this group has the authority*' or '*What would Jim think?*' exemplify this, as does the '*waver game*' where a group cycles back and forth between two or more alternative decisions without ever coming to a final decision. When they almost get there, they immediately flip back to the opposite possibility.

Paradoxically, this seeming bias for action is most likely a manifestation of the avoidance of real change, something that Schon described as '*dynamic conservatism*' – a tendency to fight hard in order to remain the same (5).

OD has often been seen as a means of enhancing organisational learning. However, OD has also been identified as an outside-in process which tends to see action learning instrumentally – viewing it as a simple tool to be used in order to achieve organisational ends. By contrast, action learning is an inside-out process, where learning is seen as valuable in and of itself. This stems from Revans' notion of the principle of insufficient mandate – that '*Those unable to change themselves cannot change what goes on around them*' (6). Action is thus seen as the **servant** of learning and serves as a motivator for it. Action is not therefore the aim of action learning, but is an input, as well as an output. So obtaining an appropriate balance between the extent that action learning is organisation-focused (with a bias for action) or individual-focused (with a bias for learning) or both is a major challenge.

There has been a tendency for action learning to focus largely on individual development and to hope that by a '*sum of the parts*' (7) or '*aggregation*' (8) effect it would lead to organisational improvement. Yet the divide between personal and organisational development is a grey area. Perhaps instead the real issue is how can personal learning and development be shared and understood organisationally? This is especially pertinent in the public services, where much of health, social and community care is located. The types of challenges which such services face are typically '*wicked*' problems (9) such as mental health, obesity or child protection, all of which cross organisational and professional boundaries. In such organisations, it is difficult (although not impossible) to justify action learning as purely a means of individual development. The emphasis instead inevitably therefore has to be on the organisation and the wider system – so not just addressing and resolving organisational problems, but also deriving and sharing collective learning from that experience through inter-connectivity and networking.

Returning to the obstetrics service example outlined in Chapter 3, where the examples of single- and double-loop learning were described, learning at the whole system level implies the necessity for learning how to learn, sometimes known as triple-loop or '*deutero-learning*' or '*meta-learning*' (10,11). In the obstetrics case the experience of refocusing obstetric services to better meet patient needs and expectations is not lost on the hospital. Structurally and culturally, the organisation encourages the transfer of such valuable lessons. Those factors that assisted such a reconfiguring (and those that impeded it) in the double-loop example are then analysed, described and communicated within the organisation. This is not done through formal written reports, but through informal communications, temporary work placements and the development of cross-service teams. Thus the obstetric service is able to share with other hospital services the lessons learned about learning to reconfigure. Triple-loop learning thus involves sharing the lessons learned from one service throughout the organisation in order to improve both single- and double-loop learning.

There is also a powerful argument which claims that action-learning facilitators in such public service organisations need to have or to develop a '*bilingual ability*' (12). This means that, in addition to exercising excellent facilitation skills, they also need to acquire a familiarity with relevant public policy language and thinking vis-à-vis the wider organisational system and to be able to identify such issues as repeating patterns of behaviour, continuing blockages to change and organisational dysfunction or '*messiness*'. In doing so, there is an onus on them to develop and share such organisational knowledge.

So what are the means by which such inter-connectivity and networking may be fostered?

- **Preparation and design:** Even before action learning is adopted within an organisation or organisations, considering the questions raised in the facilitator's checklist in Chapter 11 can be a useful way of establishing a baseline. Of particular importance is the assessment of whether the culture and climate in the organisation(s) concerned relates to the underlying ethos of action learning, as raised in Chapter 5, the key issues being:
  - Does the organisation really want to do it?
  - Is the organisation a place where it is ready to do it?

  In particular, it is important to consider whether there already exists a key group of sponsors, clients and others who can facilitate such organisational learning, and if such a group does not exist, whether it can be brought together and created. This will involve less of a focus on the '*internal*' facilitation of action learning sets and much more on the '*external*' initiation and formation processes before sets ever even meet – patient and time-consuming work on developing what has been described as a '*structure of welcome*' (13). Such work may be done by a facilitator, provided that such a person has the entrée to, and the respect of, senior people in the organisation(s) concerned. Alternatively, such a role of '*accoucheur*' or midwife who helps action learning to emerge, may be taken on by a senior organisational leader or manager. The role is close to what Schon (5) described as a '*tolkatch*' – an informal networker, middleman, broker, fixer and dealmaker.
- **Learning architecture:** This has been described as:

  > The way an organisation promotes and structures learning, both individual and organizational. (14)

Learning architecture relates to the mechanisms for sharing the learning emerging from the sets with the wider system. It is a system-wide, systematic and coordinated effort at learning and sharing good practice across the whole organisation which draws upon a whole range of different learning initiatives which historically have always been tactical in nature and aimed at specific challenges or groups of individuals. Such learning initiatives might well include action learning sets, communities of practice, focus groups, learning networks, coaching, mentoring, shadowing, secondments and large group events, such as future search conferences and open space technology (15,16). These initiatives are then linked together coherently and designed to meet organisational requirements and needs. The notion of a learning architecture is important because:

- The promotion and facilitation of both individual and organisational learning requires its own strategy and structure, from senior champions to local infrastructures.
- Without a systematic approach to developing and harnessing the learning of people in different parts of an organisation or across organisations, learning will be limited to isolated pockets or '*cultural islands*' and blocked by numerous barriers and boundaries to transmission and exchange.
- Within cybernetics the Law of Requisite Variety (17) proposes that for any system to adapt to its external environment, its internal controls and adaptive systems must incorporate the variety found in that environment. If the internal variety is reduced, then the system will be unable to cope with the external variety. So internal diversity should be welcomed and exploited and action learning sets are a vital means of fostering innovation and learning through the diversity of set membership. It has been suggested that:

> Whereas many decision-making procedures are variety-reducing in that they attempt to create a clear focus or decision domain by eliminating as much as possible, action learning seeks to create a situation that is variety-increasing. The outsider or non-expert who may only be tangentially linked to the way an issue is defined, may in the end have one of the most important ideas to contribute, by virtue of this distance and the fact that he or she is not immersed in taken-for-granted opinions. (18)

Pedler and Attwood (19), in reviewing their experience of working with action learning in NHS pathology services, concluded that a number of factors needed to be in place to ensure that the impact of action learning extended beyond the set. They were:

- The local system takes a strategic approach to the setting-up of sets and links them to other relevant activities and networks.
- Sets are aware of the wider context within which they are working, including how their organisations work, who and what they need to influence, and how best to do this.
- An influential person within the wider system takes a close and supportive interest (either by design or adoption) in what sets are doing, and helps them, where appropriate, to grapple with issues.
- Proper account is taken of the wider context of national policies and initiatives.

Likewise, Olsson et al. (20) highlighted the importance of early time and effort being devoted to trust-building across individuals and organisations and emphasised the significance of such factors as support from senior leadership and management, the modelling of openness, the need to agree on codes of conduct or rules of engagement and of meeting at a '*neutral*' venue. A local government example (21) described a series of nine '*pre-meetings*' before sets even began to operate.

Two useful examples of how linkages can be made between action learning sets and the wider organisational system and can encourage collaborative ways of working between sets and other organisational groupings are outlined below:

- Nicolini et al. (22) described attempts to link action learning to whole system change conferences. Dialogue and collective engagement was mobilised between a number of sets ('*a structure that reflects*') and large change conferences ('*a structure that connects*'), the latter being a space where reflection can be linked to power. Such a process required the active engagement of key decision makers in order to ensure success, echoing Gentle's (23) imperative for the need for senior decision makers to move beyond mere leadership and management rhetoric.

- Flowers and Reeve (24) created what they termed the '*knowledge fusion method*' which was a whole group action learning approach – '*a combination of traditional action learning and open space technology but extended beyond traditional constraints by the addition of web-based virtual communities*'.

The ultimate aim of a learning architecture will be to permanently embed the action learning process within continuing cycles of organisational review, planning and learning – to '*hard-wire*' learning into organisational systems, policies and procedures. In this respect, a useful concept is that of **absorptive or adaptive capacity** – the capacity of an organisation to acquire, assimilate and apply useful knowledge (25). Absorptive capacity is shaped by both external and internal factors. The ***external factors*** include:

- Wider environmental conditions, such as the pace of change which the organisation experiences, the scale of challenge which it encounters, and so on.
- How easy it is for the organisation to access both explicit and tacit knowledge about its performance and how that knowledge is captured, shared and used.
- How the organisation works with other stakeholders, the extent that those relationships exhibit collaboration, trust, mutual respect and parity and how close or distant they are.

The internal factors comprise:

- How inward or outward looking the organisation is – how it responds to experimentation and innovation and how hierarchical or controlling it is.
- The existence of strategies which make the focus of performance improvement clear, are shared and supported and are realistic and consistent over time.
- The existence of structures and processes for enacting knowledge mobilisation– intelligence gathering, capacity development, change management and so on.

The way that an organisation acquires, assimilates and applies knowledge (or learns) seems to be shaped by a combination of these external and internal factors (26) and action learning is potentially a key enabler in making this happen.

There can be no standard blueprint for the design of an organisational learning architecture because it will need to reflect the particular circumstances and nature of the organisation or organisations concerned, the context or setting in which they operate and the key stakeholders and partners. What is clear, however, is that it implies major change to pre-existing organisational education and training and performance management systems (27). As the nature of such a learning architecture will be both collaborative and collective, the processes by which it is designed should also be collaborative – that is, it should involve all significant stakeholders and/or partners. Unless there is such a collaborative effort, it is unlikely that the learning architecture design created will have the ownership and '*buy-in*' which will be essential for success. The danger, of course, is that organisational power and politics may serve to constrain as well as to enhance such effort and the design process needs to recognise this and plan to deal with it (28).

REFERENCES

1. P. Hind, M. Frost and S. Rowley, The resilience audit and the psychological contract, *Journal of Management Psychology* 11 (7); 1996: 18–29.
2. V. Marsick and K. Watkins, *Informal and Incidental Learning in the Workplace* (London: Routledge, 1990).
3. R. Merton, *Bureaucratic Structure and Personality in Social Theory and Social Structure* (Glencoe, IL: The Free Press, 1958).
4. J. Edmonstone, Action learning and organisation development, in *Action Learning in Practice*, Fourth edition, ed. Mike Pedler (Farnham: Gower Publishing, 2011).
5. D. Schon, *Beyond the Stable State: Public and Private Learning in a Changing Society* (Harmondsworth: Penguin, 1973).
6. R. Revans, *ABC of Action Learning* (Farnham: Gower Publishing, 2011).
7. C. Rigg, Action learning for organisational and systemic development: Towards a 'Both-And' understanding of 'I' and 'We', *Action Learning: Research & Practice* 5 (2); 2008: 105–116.
8. I. De Loo, The troublesome relationship between action learning and organisational growth, *Journal of Workplace Learning* 14 (6); 2002: 245–255.
9. H. Rittel and M. Webber, Dilemmas in a general theory of planning, *Policy Science* 4 (1); 1973: 155–163.
10. J. Biggs, The role of Meta-Learning in study process, *British Journal of Educational Psychology* 55; 1985: 185–212.
11. P. Tosey, M. Visser and M. Saunders, The origins and conceptualisations of triple loop learning: A critical review, *Management Learning* 43 (3); 2012: 291–307.
12. C. Rigg, Action learning in the public service system: Issues, tensions and a future agenda, in *Action Learning, Leadership and Organisational Development in Public Services*, ed. Clare Rigg and Sue Richards (Abingdon: Routledge, 2006), 195–206.
13. R. Revans, *The Origins and Growth of Action Learning* (Bromley: Chartwell-Bratt, 1982).
14. W. Wilhelm, *Learning Architectures: Building Individual and Organisational Learning* (New Mexico: GCA Press, 2005).
15. B. Bunker and B. Alban, *Large Group Interventions: Engaging the Whole System for Rapid Change* (San Francisco, CA: Jossey-Bass, 1997).
16. M. Weisbord and S. Janoff, *Future Search: An Action Guide to Finding Common Ground in Organisations and Communities* (San Francisco, CA: Berrett-Koehler Publishers, 1995).
17. W.R. Ashby, Requisite variety and its implications for the control of complex systems, *Cybernetica* 1 (2); 1958: 83–99.
18. G. Morgan and R. Ramirez, Action learning: A holographic metaphor for guiding social change, *Human Relations* 37 (1); 1984: 1–27.
19. M. Pedler and M. Attwood, Do action learning sets generate 'Social Capital'? *Paper Presented at 2nd International Action Learning Conference*, Henley Business School, March, 2010.
20. A. Olsson, C. Wadell, P. Odenrick and M. Bergendahl, An action learning network method for increased innovation capability in organisations, *Action Learning: Research & Practice* 7 (2); 2010: 167–179.
21. C. Yapp, Levels of action learning and holding groups to the experience, in *Action Learning, Leadership and Organisational Development in Public Services*, ed. Clare Rigg and Sue Richards (Abingdon: Routledge, 2006), 104–116.

22. D. Nicolini, M. Sher, S. Childerstone and M. Gorli, In search of the 'Structure that reflects': Promoting organisational reflection practices in A UK Health Authority, in *Organising Reflection*, eds. Mike Reynolds and Russ Vince (Aldershot: Ashgate Publishing, 2004).
23. P. Gentle, The influence on an action learning set of affective and organisational cultural factors, *Action Learning: Research & Practice* 7 (1); 2010: 17–28.
24. S. Flowers and S. Reeve, Management education and development through the application of the knowledge fusion method: A radical model to accelerate management learning, *International Journal of Management Education* 2 (3); 2002: 27–34.
25. W. Cohen and D. Levinthal, Absorptive capacity: A new perspective on learning and innovation, *Administrative Science Quarterly* 35 (1); 1990: 128–152.
26. K. Walshe, G. Harvey, C. Skelcher and P. Jas, *Could Do Better?: Knowledge, Learning and Performance Improvement in Public Services* (Manchester: Manchester Business School/University of Birmingham, 2009).
27. M. Pedler, D. Warburton, D. Wilkinson, N. Spencer and D. Wade, *Improving Poor Environments: The Role of Learning Architectures in Developing and Spreading Good Practice* (Bristol: Environment Agency, 2007).
28. T. Lawrence, M. Mauws, B. Dyck and R. Kleysen, The politics of organisational learning: Integrating power into the 4I framework, *Academy of Management Review* 30 (1); 2005: 180–191.

13

Evaluating action learning*

Faced with the choice between changing one's mind and proving that there is no need to do so, almost everybody gets busy on the proof.

(John Kenneth Galbraith)

The range of benefits that it is possible to derive from action learning are outlined in Chapter 4. Although these are largely focused at individual and organisational levels, there are clearly also some benefits to the facilitator, in terms of a deeper understanding of self, other individuals and group dynamics; improved knowledge and skill and enhanced experience in facilitation and reputation (1–4). Most accounts of action learning in practice have tended to concentrate largely on what are perceived as successful applications. Yet there can also be real value in reviewing and reflecting on those occasions when action learning is less successful and the learning which can flow from such reflection and review can offer useful insights for facilitators and organisations alike (5,6). One useful but small-scale evaluation of action learning set facilitator development programmes, for example, identified an impact on a number of key areas, including perceived skills in facilitation, critical thinking and evaluation, together with increased confidence levels in supporting colleagues. There were also reported changes in individual (and sometimes organisational) practices (7). Thus, the evaluation of action learning deserves proper attention and application.

PROBLEMS WITH EVALUATION

Traditionally, evaluations of development activities have depended largely on the impressions formed by their participants, often after the event or series of events have taken place. Such an approach makes it difficult to form an accurate impression of the real impact that a development programme may have had on its participants and on their organisations. This is partly because of the retrospective nature of such evaluations, and also due to a (perhaps inevitable) rosy glow that surrounds individual and group recollections of events through which the participants have passed.

While there is almost universal agreement on the importance and value of evaluation, the evidence also suggests that many developmental activities and processes continue to follow, one after the other, with little evaluation of their impact before organisations transition on to

* This chapter is based upon 'The challenge of evaluating action learning', *Action Learning: Research & Practice* 12 (2); 2015: 131–145.

the next activity (8). This is particularly true in parts of the public sector, where national initiatives are often *'cascaded'* in a hierarchical manner down into local settings and where evaluation of the success, or otherwise, of such initiatives is particularly rare, perhaps because such evaluation might result in an *'unacceptable finding'* which could potentially be career-limiting for those associated with the evaluation.

In seeking to evaluate any developmental activity it is relatively easy to collect data on:

- **Reactions:** To an event or events in the form of individual thoughts and feelings. This is the level of the *'happy sheet'* administered to a captive audience at the end of an event and is the most common form of assessment used. It is slightly more difficult, though not impossible, to also collect data on.
- **Learning:** That is, to what degree participants acquire or change the intended knowledge, skills and attitudes, based upon their participation in the event. It is even more problematic to collect data on resulting changes in their performance.
- **Behaviour:** In other words, to what degree participants actually apply what they have learned when they are back in their job and organisational setting. Finally, it is very difficult indeed to collect data on.
- **Outcomes or results:** To what degree targeted outcomes occur as a result of the event and subsequent reinforcement – in other words the impact or effect of changed behaviour on organisational performance (9).

The movement from reactions to outcomes evaluation introduces a significant number of intervening variables (other things happening to the individual and/or going on in the organisation) which make it more difficult (some would even say impossible) to ascribe a simple cause-and-effect relationship. Moreover, the correlation between the levels is weak – a positive result at one level does not necessarily lead to a positive result at the next. By concentrating on the (relatively easy to assess) participant reactions, the tendency is thus to sideline those contextual factors that might affect both the event and its impact.

Moreover, development activity such as action learning works much more through **generative causation** (i.e. creating those conditions where things can change and move on to destinations as yet unknown) as through **successionist causation** (i.e. achieving predictable and pre-known outcomes) (10).

A further approach to evaluation of learning is the Return on Investment (ROI) methodology (11) developed from the 1980s. Its key feature is the calculation of the monetary value of investing in a programme. The results of a programme are converted into a financial value, enabling a cost-benefit analysis to take place. Those programme results which cannot be monetised are called *'intangibles'* and in the ROI approach have a secondary importance. In ROI only financial quantitative data really matters and *'intangibles'*, as evidenced by qualitative data, are relegated to a secondary role. This approach therefore risks either minimising such results or forcing an essentially hypothetical and subjective financial value on them. Yet such *'intangibles'* can, of course, lead to significant organisational benefits over time.

Although these are major problems with evaluation, there are also others, including the following:

- ***Time***: How to evaluate development interventions over the short term that are intended to have much longer-term impacts? One possible approach suggested is that of *'intermediate measurement'* or assessment of distance travelled so far towards an ultimate intended destination.

- ***Complexity***: As previously mentioned, where there are potentially multiple intervening variables, how can the effect of one activity be disentangled from the others, particularly when they may overlap? One response may be to conclude that it is not possible to identify causality conclusively, or perhaps only at the individual, rather than the organisational, level.
- ***Value***: What actually counts as '*success*'? What is valued and by whom? Recent approaches typically address this issue by including all the key stakeholders in the evaluation process and seeking to surface the assumptions behind activities – what exactly are people seeking to do through them?
- ***Horse for courses***: The size and complexity of the evaluation need to be in proportion to the activity being evaluated and the form the evaluation takes should, in turn, reflect the values underlying the activity or programme itself (12).
- ***Cost***: To conduct evaluation is not cost-free. While clients of developmental activity are rightly concerned with outcomes, evaluation will entail additional work, with its inherent costs, whether this is sourced internally or externally. Ideally, such evaluation (and the associated costs) would be planned into the development programme at the outset, although in practice this seldom happens and evaluation is often conducted as an afterthought.
- ***Politics***: Evaluation is a complex and highly political process. The underlying assumption behind evaluation is that discovering '*what works*' is desirable because it will result in evidence-based future action. However, policy decisions regarding developmental activity can, and often are, made despite the evidence of what does or does not work in practice. Evaluation can even be designed to gather data that support a particular policy direction – policy-based evidence, rather than evidence-based policy. If evaluation results are sensitive politically then they may even never be released publicly and may be ignored. Decisions are made based upon much more than evidence – values, interests, personalities, timing, circumstance and happenstance all also play their parts.

> You don't pull up radishes to see how they are growing.
>
> *(Anonymous)*

One alternative suggestion made (13) is to rely on the processes of informal evaluation that occur continually at all levels of an organisation. Rather than emphasising systematic and planned measurement, it is suggested that the key may lie in focusing on processes that facilitate and encourage dialogue across professional, managerial and organisational boundaries: the pooling of experiences and informal assessment that have the potential to lead to shared learning. This can appear an attractive approach as it has been pointed out (14) that quantitative measurement may not just be undesirable for certain activities, but perhaps impossible. To measure anything an objective yardstick is needed – such as centimetres for length, kilogrammes for weight and litres for volume. Human activity at work involves a range of complex tasks that are highly context-dependent and it may well be a fallacy to believe that such an activity can be measured objectively using a yardstick and resulting in '*hard*' figures. Verhaeghe notes that measurement of this kind tends to use Likert scales, which involve respondents rating statements by selecting from a range of possible responses (such as poor, adequate, good and very good) or figures (often as −2, −1, 0, +1, and +2). These are intuitive approximations based on subjective criteria, and any translation of results into figures serves to create a false impression of objective quantifiability. Such a process has also been described as methodologically specious. It is claimed, for example, that the OFSTED inspection regime for schools in

England is marked by words which do not mean what they say they mean. '*Outstanding*' for example, really means '*Everyone should be this*'; '*Good*' really means '*No better than you ought to be*' and everything below that simply means '*Awful*' (15). The danger of making such decisions based solely on quantitative observations and ignoring all others is sometimes known as the '*McNamara Fallacy*', named after Robert McNamara, the US Secretary of Defence during the Vietnam War. It runs as follows:

> The first step is to measure whatever can be easily measured. This is OK as far as it goes. The second step is to disregard what can't be measured easily or to give it an arbitrary value. This is artificial and misleading. The third step is to presume that whatever can't be measured easily really isn't important. This is blindness. The fourth step is to say whatever can't be measured easily really doesn't exist. This is suicide. (16)

The underlying assumption of such approaches would seem to be that everything in organisational life is driven by some form of competition and that such competition can only be fostered by constant measurement and comparison. In their major review of evaluation for leadership and management development, Hirsh et al. (8) unsurprisingly therefore recommend the combining of both quantitative and qualitative data.

PROBLEMS WITH EVALUATING ACTION LEARNING

If there are major difficulties in evaluating developmental activities in general, these seem to be even greater when consideration is given to evaluating action learning. As previously noted, action learning is now accepted as comprising both ethos and method, but evaluation typically tends to focus only on action learning as method. If the general culture of an organisation or set of organisations does not match or favour the underlying action learning ethos, then action learning can, as a result, seem to be a counter-cultural '*island*' and so can be easily dismissed. The notion of a cultural '*envelope*' which may be more or less developmental and supportive of action learning has been advanced (6) and supports the need for a degree of '*fit*' between the ethos of action learning and the organisational culture(s).

Chapter 5 indicated that action learning can address both '*tame*' and '*wicked*' problems, but is particularly pertinent to the latter. Concentration on tame problems means that evaluation is inevitably restricted to Levels 1 and 2 of the locus of an action learning set's work, where Level 1 is devoted simply to problem-solving and the implementation of solutions in relation to a specific and well-defined problem and Level 2 not only encompasses Level 1 but also includes reframing of the problem and the conscious transfer of skills from the original problem situation to another. It precludes considerations at Levels 3 and 4, where Level 3 embodies both Levels 1 and 2 plus personal development, self-knowledge and an understanding of personal learning styles and processes and Level 4 encompasses the previous three levels plus a focus on organisational culture and transformation in relation to life/career issues. Levels 3 and 4 are most likely where '*wicked*' problems are located (17).

A further difficulty lies with the open-ended and unpredictable nature of action learning processes. It is difficult, probably even impossible, to predict specific outcomes from action learning in advance and in detail. The starting or presenting problem that a set member arrives with may change or evolve from interactions and dialogue with other set members and with the facilitator. The challenges which set members encounter may be unexpected and highly individual in nature. Set members may experience insight into their own behaviour or the culture of their organisations that stimulate actions which were not predictable prior to the set being formed. Even when the implications of using action learning have been clearly explained within an organisation, the system is not always ready for the repercussions which spill out of the set members working on their issues. Action learning is thus quite unlike more conventional '*training*' approaches, which seek to constrain uncertainty and aim to establish order through curricula, best practices and set techniques (18), and is instead marked by a high degree of emergent learning.

A related difficulty for evaluation of action learning lies with the potential multiplicity of stakeholders. Each individual set member may have different intentions with regard to the set and the problem or problems which they bring to it, and these perceptions may change over the set's duration. While some set members might be self-directed volunteers and some sets might be completely self-organised, in the majority of cases where action learning programmes are intra-organisationally or inter-organisationally based, this is unlikely to be the case. With such programmes each set member will also have a sponsor – an immediate line manager or senior professional colleague who will have expectations derived from what they have personally experienced of action learning or have heard about it – or not. In one example, for instance:

> The sponsoring managers did not really understand what action learning was – they had never experienced it themselves and had never attended an event where it was explained to them. They did not really know what the commitment to doing action learning entailed and were therefore not fully signed up to it. In deciding who to sponsor on the programme they were not making an informed choice – rather it was a "box-ticking" response. (6)

Set members will hopefully also have a senior organisational champion or champions who have enabled action learning to take place and they will have a perception of the purpose of an action learning programme, as will the facilitator. All these stakeholders will have varying levels of experience and understanding of action learning and therefore different expectations of outcomes.

It has been suggested (19) that action learning can make a significant contribution to the development of social capital. Social capital is collective capacity or efficacy – the quantity and quality of the relational connections within or across any organisation, network or system. It exists in the active connections among people where trust, mutual understanding and shared values make cooperative action possible. Seeking to evaluate the quantity and quality of such interpersonal and inter-group relationships is a major challenge to the field of evaluation research.

Finally, there is the question of what kind of action learning it is intended to evaluate. Chapter 3 outlined the variety of approaches available.

> Not everything that counts can be counted, and not everything that can be counted counts.
>
> *(William Bruce Cameron)*

TOWARDS A WAY FORWARD

A first step can be to distinguish between two different types of evaluation. Some evaluation is **formative** (or developmental). It is concerned with making things better, with steering and improving the process of action learning while it is happening. It serves to reinforce learning by using evaluation as a contribution to the learning process itself. Other evaluation is **summative** (or judgemental) and is concerned with assessing the overall measurable impact or contribution of action learning (20). The two evaluation approaches can be presented as '*ideal types*' for the purposes of comparison, as shown in Figure 13.1. Summative evaluation is more likely to be valued by budget holders, to rely on '*hard*' data and to require quick answers. Formative evaluation is more likely to be favoured by the developers, who value the rich information accrued, including the impact of context or setting on learning and performance.

In practice, evaluation of action learning needs to adopt both formative and summative approaches. Formative (within-set) evaluation should be part of the ongoing work of each set meeting and some of the tools identified in Part 3 of this book can be helpful here. Additionally, and on a more informal basis, there can be value in reviewing ground-rules, set members' views on the set process and the balance between support and challenge and action and reflection. Set members might, for example, retrospectively score themselves at the beginning of the action learning programme and then at the end in order to benchmark change. Emergent as well as predicted outcomes might be included. Additionally, set members might also evaluate what ongoing organisational factors impinged on their actions. The focus throughout is on evaluating progress with learning and with reviewing the helpful, and less helpful, norms of the set, with the intention of making future set meetings more productive.

The greater challenge comes with summative evaluation. Drawing on a major national review of evaluation of leadership and management development (8) and an examination of evaluations of eight major leadership development programmes in the National Health Service in the UK (12), a summative evaluation framework for action learning is proposed, based on a series of questions under seven headings.

	Formative evaluation	Summative evaluation
Goal	Understanding and perspective	Truth and scientific acceptance
Measurement	Qualitative data	Quantitative data
Evaluator approach	Subjectivity	Objectivity
Relationships	Closeness and involvement	Distance and detachment
Inquiry mode	Induction	Deduction
Outcomes	Context-bound	Generalisations

Figure 13.1 Formative and summative evaluation.

Purpose

- What particular variant of action learning is being used, and therefore evaluated?
- How exactly is action learning being used – as an activity interwoven with other aspects of a programme; as a discrete development activity in its own right or as a link between a formal programme and the workplace?
- What exactly do we want to know about the programme?
- Who are the key stakeholders? What are their expectations of the programme?
- What do they believe it is seeking to do?
- Is there clarity over the intended purpose and anticipated outcomes and benefits from the programme, both individually and organisationally? Are these short-term or long-term?
- Are the personal and organisational development needs the programme is intended to address articulated? Are they clear? Are such needs retrospective or prospective?

Fit

- To what extent is there '*fit*' between the values underpinning the programme and the culture(s) of the participants' organisations, or with attempts to change them?
- Is there clarity of the underlying assumptions of the programme with regard to the nature of adult learning?

Preparation and support

- Is there clarity regarding the respective roles of set members, facilitator(s), sponsors, champions, and so on? Are these expectations explicit or implicit? Are they available as a reference point, if needed, across the duration of the programme?
- Are there recognised organisational champions for the programme? Who are they? What is the nature of their support in practical and symbolic terms? Is it sustained across and beyond the programme's duration?
- How clear are set members' sponsors about the nature of action learning and the demands it is likely to make on them, on the set member and on the organisation?
- Do local development staff see it as part of their role to support set members before, during and after the programme? Do they have the competence, motivation and time to do so?
- Are there in place appropriate '*entry strategies*' to prepare set members for their involvement in the programme and the level of challenge and support that they may expect from set membership, and also '*re-entry strategies*' for the transition back into work, where the level of support and challenge is unlikely to resemble that encountered in the set?

Membership

- Is participation in the programme voluntary or directed? If directed, what are the internal organisational selection criteria for set membership? To what extent (if at all) is there competition for membership of the programme?
- To what extent is biographical and other data relevant to the evaluation, such as:
    - Gender of set members
    - Age range of set members
    - Professional/occupational background of set members

- Level of seniority in the organisation of set members
- Length of time in the present post
- Previous experience of action learning
- Frequency of set meetings
- Duration of set meetings
- Participation rate of set members across the set meetings

Issues

- Is the focus of the issues which set members bring to the set on tame or wicked problems or both?
- How much choice or prescription is there for set members in deciding on tame or wicked problems?
- Who is doing the deciding? (This particularly relates to business-driven action learning where there might not necessarily always be congruence between what the organisation deems to be an appropriate problem to work on and that preferred by the set member.)

Steering

- Are there in place effective arrangements for steering the programme across its duration and for reviewing and modifying it where necessary?
- How much flexibility is there in programme design terms? Can in-programme, real-time changes be easily made?

Evaluation process

- Who is the evaluation information for?
- When will the evaluation information be needed?
- In what form will evaluation information be needed?
- How will evaluation information be collected and analysed? By whom?
- What will the '*product*' of the evaluation process be?
- What are the costs or resource implications of the evaluation, in time and money terms?
- Will the benefits of the evaluation outweigh the costs of undertaking it?
- Will the evaluation contribute to an evidence-base of '*what works, in what circumstances and why?*' Will it move matters forward?

This framework offers a fairly pragmatic means of evaluating action learning and would involve the collection and analysis of both hard and soft data. What it does not necessarily do is to establish a clear causal link between involvement in an action learning programme and desirable personal and organisational outcomes. The only way to accomplish this might be to adopt a '*counter-factual*' approach (21). This approach would involve evaluators who were not aware of, or associated with, the action learning programme being used to investigate participating organisations in a carefully choreographed blind manner in order to ascertain:

- ***What has happened?*** What kind of individual and organisational changes or improvements had recently taken place?
- ***How did it happen and who was involved?*** What changed behaviour and activity had been exhibited in delivering these changes or improvements?

- ***What changes had been achieved and whether they were sustainable?*** Whether these changes or improvements could be linked directly to the action learning programme?

However, the logistics of such an approach are complex and the potential costs of undertaking an evaluation along such lines would be highly likely to outweigh the potential benefits.

Communicating the evaluation results can be seen as a process which is itself evaluative. For example, at the end of a programme, senior stakeholders (Champions) may meet set members to hear about their learning and their actions and, if there is a willingness, such senior stakeholders could invite set members' insights into other related organisational issues. In this way evaluation becomes a more dynamic process leading to further change and influence, rather than simply resulting in a report.

The extent to which an action learning programme delivers recognisable personal and organisational benefits depends, of course, to a major degree on the extent to which the culture of the organisation(s) concerned are welcoming and supportive. The major evaluation study of leadership and management development programmes (8) concluded that implementation of change was most likely when:

- There was a fit between the development approach being used and the corporate culture, or as part of a strategy to change it.
- There were regular opportunities for standing back from work and reflecting.
- There were continuing opportunities for networking with colleagues in similar roles or facing similar challenges.

There is clearly no '*magic bullet*' approach to the evaluation of action learning. The best advice may be that from the above-mentioned study:

> Adopt a cheerful spirit of enquiry rather than the leaden heart which comes from seeing evaluation as a difficult chore.

Moreover, evaluation does not remove the need for the exercise of judgement. A survey which sought to identify learning from evaluation studies in health care concluded:

> Evaluation can only ever provide good quality information to inform decision-making. It is unlikely to supply ready-made answers because the results will need to be interpreted as part of a process of discussion and judgement, with the views of different stakeholders and the intended outcomes of the activity being taken into account. (22)

> Life is lived forward, but understood backward.
>
> *(Soren Keirkegaard)*

REFERENCES

1. G. Weiland and H. Leigh, *Changing Hospitals: A Report on the Hospital Internal Communications Project* (London: Tavistock Publications, 1971).
2. G. Weiland and A. Bradford, An evaluation of the hospital internal communications project, in *Improving Health Care Management*, eds. George Weiland and Alan Bradford (Ann Arbor, MI: Health Administration Press, 1981).

3. G. Wills and C. Oliver, Measuring the return on investment from management action learning, *Management Development Review* 9 (1); 1996: 17–21.
4. L. Beaty, *Action Learning*, Learning & Teaching Support Network CPD Paper 1, 2003.
5. J. Oliver, Reflections on a failed action learning intervention, *Action Learning: Research & Practice* 5 (1): 79–83.
6. J. Edmonstone, When action learning doesn't "Take": Reflections on the DALEK programme, *Action Learning: Research & Practice* 7 (1); 2010: 89–97.
7. C. Abbott, L. Burtney and C. Wall, Building capacity in social care: An evaluation of a national programme of action learning facilitator development, *Action Learning: Research & Practice* 10 (2); 2013: 168–177.
8. W. Hirsh, P. Tamkin, V. Garrow and J. Burgoyne, *Evaluating Management and Leadership Development: New Ideas and Practical Approaches* (Brighton: Institute for Employment Studies, 2011).
9. D. Kirkpatrick and J. Kirkpatrick, *Evaluating Training Programs: The Four Levels*, Fourth edition (San Francisco, CA: Berrett-Koehler, 1998).
10. R. Pawson and N. Tilley, *Realistic Evaluation* (London: Sage, 1997).
11. J. Phillips and P. Phillips, *The Basics of ROI* www.humanresourcesiq.com/hr-technology/columns/the-basics-of-roi/, 2008.
12. J. Edmonstone, Healthcare leadership: Learning from evaluation, *Leadership in Health Services* 26 (2); 2013: 148–158.
13. D. Skinner, Evaluation and change management: Rhetoric and reality, *Human Resource Management Journal* 14 (3); 2004: 5–19.
14. P. Verhaeghe, *What About Me?: The Struggle for Identity in a Market-Based Society* (London: Scribe Publications, 2014).
15. Z. Williams, The entire schools inspection culture is the problem, *Guardian*, 20 October; 2014.
16. D. Yankelovich, *Corporate Priorities: A Continuing Study of the New Demands on Business* (Stanford, CT: Daniel Yankelovich Inc, 1972).
17. L. Yorks, J. O'Neil and V. Marsick, Action learning: Theoretical bases and varieties of practice, in *Action Learning: Successful Strategies for Individual, Team and Organisation Development*, eds. L. Yorks, J. O'Neil and V. Marsick (Baton Rouge, LA: Academy of Human Resources Management, 1999), 1–18.
18. M. Pedler and C. Abbott, *Facilitating Action Learning: A Practitioner's Guide* (Maidenhead: Open University Press, 2013).
19. M. Pedler and M. Attwood, Do action learning sets generate 'Social capital'? *Paper Presented at 2nd International Action Learning Conference*, Henley Business School, March 2010.
20. M. Easterby-Smith, *Evaluating Management Development, Training and Education* (Aldershot: Gower, 1994).
21. J. Hardacre, R. Cragg, J. Shapiro, P. Spurgeon and H. Flanagan, *'What's Leadership Got To Do With It?': Exploring Links between Quality Improvement and Leadership in The NHS* (London: ORCNI Ltd for the Health Foundation, 2011).
22. L. Larsen, J. Cummins and H. Brown, *Learning from Evaluation: Summary of Reports of Evaluations of Leadership Initiatives* (London: Office for Public Management/NHS Leadership Centre, 2005).

14

Postscript: Action learning as reflective activism

What we think, or what we know, or what we believe is, in the end, of little consequence. The only consequence is what we do.

(John Ruskin)

If the little that we know about the future is that we do not know much about it, then a key responsibility of anyone who is concerned with personal and organisational development is not just to provide people with tools that may be out-of-date before they have even been fully mastered, but rather to help them to become confident and competent designers and makers of their own learning as they go along. Another analogy is that people increasingly need to become their own map-makers and not just the readers and interpreters of others' maps.

In all walks of life, new and better ways of doing things can be discovered only if experiment and diversity are permitted, are welcomed and are fostered. The success of such experiments cannot, of course, be guaranteed in advance, so innovators must have some scope for getting things wrong without being punished for it. This scope is what engineers term '*redundancy*' – the capability to deal with unlikely eventualities. Creating such redundant capacity means allowing the space for diversity and experiment, much of which may possibly be wasted, but without which new eventualities cannot even be encouraged to emerge. An action learning set is, of course, just such a potential space.

In the current times of increased inequality and insecurity in the larger society there is, for many people, a strong sense of powerlessness abroad – a belief that nothing can be done to change the situation in which people find themselves. Action learning is the antithesis of this belief. It is almost a therapeutic process in that it helps people to take a more active orientation towards life in general and to overcome this dominant tendency to think, feel and be passive towards the pressures of life, but rather to embrace the opportunities and challenges of organisational and social change. It demonstrates its worth in terms of the capacities it creates for intelligent action, rather than in terms of its contribution to formal knowledge, as it creates conditions that are always evolving and are open-ended.

We must be the change we wish to see in the world.

(Mahatma Ghandi)

Action learning serves to cultivate what has been described as '*reflective activism*' (1) or '*practical authoring*' (2) – a stance that encourages us to own the processes by which we and others construct and sustain our worlds. It encourages us all (leaders, managers, professionals and others) to engage in reflective practice. Such practice includes the application of relevant knowledge within the workplace and beyond in order to inform and to enhance our actions. It requires our active engagement in a continual review and repositioning of our assumptions, values and practice. As such, it requires a thorough understanding of oneself and of the values and moral purpose that underpin our personal and professional practice – in other words, a journey of self-discovery. The knowledge created by such engagement is relevant to the specific contexts in which we work and live and to the specific individuals with whom we work – our colleagues, employees, patients, clients and so on (3). It is a form of '*artistry in practice*' – a fluid approach in which the practitioner becomes a '*knowledgeable doer*' (4).

If we accept that '*to some extent we are all prisoners trapped within the perceptual frameworks that determine how we view our experiences*' (5), it has been claimed that, in order to stimulate our learning, we should work to apply different perspectives to what we know or assume. To enable this, Brookfield developed his 'four-lens' model in order to identify these key perspectives. He proposed that they were:

- **The autobiographical lens:** Framed by our own life experiences as individual learners and, as such, this lens can potentially be restrictive and may not consider other '*blind spots*', such as our ability to learn in modes different from our dominant one. Action learning's characterisation of this particular lens is our personal mind-set or mental model.
- **The colleagues/peers lens:** Dialogue with colleagues who experience similar situations to us but may use alternative approaches and see things differently can enable the gaining of an empathic perspective. Such dialogue engages us at the edge of our current understanding. This lens represents a significant major strength of action learning.
- **The theoretical/literature lens:** The results of research and exploration in the particular field in which we work.
- **The student lens:** A focus on the learner's viewpoint, gained through feedback, evaluation and so on.

To this, Hanson (6) has added a fifth **socio-cultural** lens which supports a wider perspective and also serves to filter the other lenses. It is determined by two aspects – the socio-cultural influence of the reflecting learner and the socio-cultural influences of the particular context in which reflection takes place. From this, Hanson defines reflective practice as:

> an active engagement in continual review and repositioning of assumptions, values and practice in the light of evaluation of multiple perspectives, including the wider socio-cultural perspectives influencing the context; transforming and transcending self and practice in order to effect change and improvement.

and suggests that such reflective practice:

- Is stimulated by a natural disposition to be curious
- Involves a complex interaction between the individual and the particular context in which they work
- Involves engaging actively with the complexities and challenges within a diverse profession or occupation

- Involves a proactive stance in all aspects of reflective thinking, learning and action, whereby individuals question, examine and challenge a range of different positions, including their own
- Is perceived as a '*way of being*' for individuals and communities of practice and that it builds upon a strong value base that assumes personal and professional responsibility for improving the quality of services
- Should be both critical and meaningful and avoid a narrow interpretation that reviews reflective practice only for external demands
- Recognises the significance of a reflexive approach which involves critical examination and '*theorisation*' of what you do and why, in relation to the impact this has upon self and others
- Requires a full critical evaluation of evidence gained from multi-dimensional reflections, including the fifth socio-cultural lens

Put another way, reflective activism maintains that '*I can at least make one person's worth of difference in the world.*' (7) and, at heart, this is action learning's ultimate credo. In commenting on Revans' overarching purpose, Willis claimed that he:

> saw plainly that each individual alive is affected by the clarity or dimness of our human insights. He thought it must take an egalitarian, self-organised effort of countless individuals in small groups to move institutions and societies in more collaborative and co-beneficial directions. More than this, it would take willingness to admit that we are all ignorant of the ways in which even quite simple problems interlock with one another and cause unbearable complications. Unravelling complexities takes more than fast-track personalities, infinite computer capabilities and fierce competitiveness. It takes patient, persistent, even sacrificial human endeavour – individuals united in common effort – because so many options we must consider are matters for the human heart to act upon. (8)

> *The world is a dangerous place to live; not because of the people who are evil, but because of the people who don't do anything about it.*
>
> *(Albert Einstein)*

REFERENCES

1. G. Morgan and R. Ramirez, Action learning: A holographic metaphor for guiding social change, *Human Relations* 37 (1); 1984: 1–27.
2. J. Shotter, *Conversational Realities: Constructing Life Through Language* (Thousand Oaks, CA: Sage, 1993).
3. K. Hanson and K. Appleby, Reflective practice, in *A Critical Companion to Early Childhood* eds. Michael Reed and Rosie Walker (London: Sage, 2014).
4. N. Thompson and J. Pascal, Developing critically reflective practice, *Reflective Practice* 13 (2); 2012: 1–15.
5. S. Brookfield, *Becoming a Critically Reflective Teacher* (San Francisco, CA: Jossey-Bass, 1995).
6. K. Hanson, *How can I support early childhood undergraduate students to develop reflective dispositions?* Ed.D thesis (Exeter University, 2012).

7. I. McGill and L. Beaty, *Action Learning: A Practitioner's Guide*, Second edition (Abingdon: Routledge, 2001).
8. V. Willis, Digging deeper: Foundations of Revans' gold standard of action learning, in *Action Learning in Practice*, Fourth edition, ed. Mike Pedler (Farnham: Gower Publishing, 2011), 71–80.

PART 3

Resources

15

What resource tools are available to help me in working in action learning?

Four different sets of resource tools are described here. The first few are personal exercises which can be worked on by individual action set members. The second group are ways of using the ongoing dynamic of the set itself. The third group of tools relate to working on the problem, issue or challenge which the set member brings to the set and continues to address in the workplace. There is a multiplicity of the latter, so a selection of those most relevant has been made. The final group of tools are useful for reviewing the set's processes and progress and are therefore helpful for formative evaluation purposes. Useful sources of other tools can be found as follows:

- Maggie Havergal and John Edmonstone, *The Facilitator's Toolkit*, Second edition (Aldershot: Gower Publishing, 2003)
- Christine Hogan, *Practical Facilitation: A Toolkit of Techniques* (London: Kogan Page, 2003)
- Becky Malby and Martin Fischer, *Tools for Change: An Invitation to Dance* (Chichester: Kingsham Press, 2006)
- And at a number of websites, such as: www.theknowledgebiz/resources/A-Guide-to-Action-Learning-along-with-Tools-and-Techniques.pdf
- www.odi.org/sites/odi.org.uk/files/odi-assets/publications-opinion-files/188.pdf

All tools are considered under the headings of:

What is it?
Why would I use it?
When would I use it?
How would I use it?

PERSONAL EXERCISES FOR INDIVIDUAL SET MEMBERS

These exercises tend to be highly meaningful to people who are in mid-career, who are contemplating a major career or life change or who have seldom been introspective about their own lifestyle and career pattern, but now wish to take stock in order to move on to the next stage in their life and/or career. It should be entirely voluntary whether individual set members do opt to undertake such work involving these exercises.

Core process exercise

What is it? This exercise is a form of biography work.

Why would I use it? It offers a way for individuals to review their existence in ways that transcend the narrow and ahistorical snapshots that many analytical approaches embody. It produces an enriched perspective which brings both the past and possible alternative futures together with the present for the purposes of understanding and action.

When would I use it? To support people seeking to place job or career problems in an overall life context.

How would I use it?

1. Divide your life into four or five sections, from birth to the present day.
2. Recall those moments, the feelings, sensations and experiences which were really fulfilling and motivating – the times of feeling at one with oneself and with the world.
3. Identify the special qualities, important patterns and themes which were around at the time of these moments.
4. From this activity, is it possible to identify the core process or processes that have run through career and/or life itself and which should be translated into the future?

Life goals exercise

What is it? This exercise is a form of biography work.

Why would I use it? It offers a way for individuals to review their existence in ways that transcend the narrow and ahistorical snapshots that many analytical approaches embody. It produces an enriched perspective which brings the past and possible futures together with the present for the purposes of understanding and action.

When would I use it? To support people seeking to place job or career problems in a life context.

How would I use it?

1. Draw an individual lifeline where one dimension (horizontal) is the passage of time from birth to the present and the other (vertical) relates to feelings of self-esteem, ranging from low to high.
2. Prepare a life inventory of important personal '*happenings*', including:
   a. Any peak experiences that can be identified
   b. Things that you know you do well
   c. Things that you know you do poorly
   d. Things that you would like to stop doing
   e. Things that you would like to do well
   f. Peak experiences that you would like to have
   g. Values that you want to live
   h. Things that you would like to start doing now

EXERCISES USING THE SET'S DYNAMICS

These exercises employ the dynamic of the set in order to illustrate specific aspects of set membership and the learning that can be derived from it.

Action learning constellations

What is it? An exercise which helps set members to visualise how close or distant work relationships are and to envisage a better alternative.
Why would I use it? To help to illustrate, in a spatial sense, the closeness or distance of work relationships.
When would I use it? When a set member describes a seemingly intractable work-based inter-relationship problem.
How would I use it?

1. The set member presenting an issue or problem describes the context, the different stakeholders involved and the related inter-relationship challenges.
2. When this is completed the set member '*places*' the other set members around the room in a constellation in order to represent the positions that those stakeholders currently occupy at that stage of the problem. Some will therefore be close to the set member, whereas others will be further apart.
3. In turn, these '*proxy stakeholders*' describe how it feels to be so positioned.
4. The presenting set member then moves the proxy stakeholders to the position which the presenter feels would be most helpful in helping to address the issue.
5. Once again, the proxy stakeholders say how the new positions feel.
6. Finally, the presenter considers the implications of these movements in the room and addresses how he or she might make them '*for real*' back in the problem situation.

Break-space exercise

What is it? An exercise designed to '*jump start*' the reflection process in action learning sets.
Why would I use it? To encourage a reflective frame of mind at the beginning of a set meeting or when tension surfaces within the set.
When would I use it? Either at the commencement of a set meeting or when matters become pressurised in the set. In the latter case, such reflection can serve to relieve the stress level and to provide positive reinforcement for the purpose of the set.
How would I use it? The facilitator suggests that set members take about 10 minutes at the start of each set meeting where all set members close their eyes, remain silent and reflect. Reflection can either be general or focused – for example, '*What is the most important thing that has happened to you since the set last met? Why is it so important? What might you learn from it?*'

For some set members, this may seem a distraction from the business of progress-reporting of their problem or issue, but it is probably also attributable to the awkwardness of being asked to reflect.

Establishing ground rules

What is it? Early in the life of the set there is a need to establish ground rules or a code of conduct to govern the behaviour of set members and the facilitator; to allay any anxieties that people may have about what might happen in the set and to establish and model shared responsibility and joint working between the set members and the facilitator.

Why would I use it? So that set members do not become disappointed or frustrated by the behaviour of the other members of the set.

When would I use it? At the first set meeting. Ground rules should be considered as provisional and open to change. They may be revisited and revised at later set meetings in order to consider whether or not they are still relevant.

How would I use it? Ground rules are of two types – practical and behavioural:

Practical:

- The life-expectancy of the set – for how long will it continue to meet?
- The frequency and duration of set meetings – how often will the set meet and for how long on each occasion?
- The format of set meetings and how time will be allocated within them, including breaks
- Attendance and punctuality at set meetings
- Declaration of any conflicts of interest by set members
- The use of jargon or abbreviations
- Note-taking – who owns the notes and what happens to any notes taken
- Each person to have roughly equal voice and time

Behavioural:

- Confidentiality – what does this actually mean in practice?
- Commitment and priority – this involves self-discipline by set members and support by their sponsoring manager/professional colleague
- Respect for and between each other
- Being non-judgemental
- Being responsible for self
- Openness
- Only one person speaks at a time
- Using 'I', not 'We' or 'One' or 'You' or 'They'
- Supporting and challenging each other
- The right to say 'No' or to decline to respond to a question or challenge

Listening in the corner exercise

What is it? An exercise which enables set members to practice reflecting on a situation by stepping away from it and looking at how others tackle it.

Why would I use it? It is most useful when only one or two set members are *'in the spotlight'* during a day or half-day meeting.

When would I use it? When there is little evidence of listening behaviour in the set or where set members experience difficulty in avoiding the *'expert'* role.

How would I use it? (Note: All suggested timings are indicative only)

1. The set member with the issue or problem that they are struggling with describes the problem to the others. The other set members listen, do not interrupt and take notes about whatever comes to mind as they listen, in particular focusing on what might lie *'underneath'* the story being told, and also on what it evokes in terms of their own feelings and associations. (*15 minutes*)

2. The set members quickly rehearse their immediate thoughts and feelings. The set member with the issue stays silent while the others are speaking, but is given the opportunity, when they are finished, to return to anything that he/she thinks significant (preferably without defence or correction). Questions for clarification may also be asked at this point, provided they are not leading questions designed to suggest a solution. (*15 minutes*)
3. The set member with the problem is invited to move out of the group and away from the others and to sit in the corner of the room – within earshot, but out of eyeshot. They should feel perfectly free to take notes on what they see and think about what happens. The other set members discuss the issue that has been '*handed over*' and the presenter's involvement in it, as if he/she was not even in the room. The aim is for them to play around with it, to explore what is going on and to reflect on their thoughts and feelings about the issue. (*30 minutes*)
4. The presenter re-joins the group to use the time as he/she wishes – to pick up on certain points, to ask for more information, to rehearse what might happen if particular proposals are carried through, and so on. The presenter might also usefully comment on:
   a. What aspects of the dialogue which they overheard that they found most interesting, thought-provoking and helpful
   b. What aspects they found most challenging and difficult
   c. What new insights have been generated
   d. What they intend to do next (*15 minutes*)
5. The set members (including the presenter) say what they have gained from the session. (*5 minutes*)

Miracle question

What is it? A method for helping a set member to describe their preferred future.

Why would I use it? When a set member seems lost in the intricacies of their problem situation with no obvious '*way out*'.

When would I use it? When a set member has some difficulty in expressing exactly what a desirable future state would look like.

How would I use it? The facilitator says to the set member '*Suppose you went to bed tonight and a miracle happened. You have absolutely no idea how it occurred, but it just did. When you wake up in the morning the issue that you have brought here to the set has gone. What will you notice that tells you that the miracle has occurred? What else?*' (Repeat this question five times) '*Who else will notice?*' '*What will they notice?*' (Repeat this five times)

Shuffled cards

What is it? An exercise designed to provide feedback anonymously to set members in order to enhance trust and safety.

Why would I use it? In order to foster a sense of safety and security within the set.

When would I use it? Early in the life of the set – possibly at the first meeting.

How would I use it? The facilitator hands three small blank filing cards times the number of set members plus themselves to each person and asks them to record on each of the three cards one positive thing – a word or a short phrase – about each person in the set. If there are, for example, five set members plus the facilitator, then each person should have 15 cards with one attribute per card. On the other side of each card set members are asked to print the name of the person the attribute applies to. The cards are not signed by the authors. The cards are placed in the centre of the set meeting, name side up, and shuffled. Each person in the set is then given their cards name-side up. Each set member may say how they feel if they wish to – but not to ask who wrote what.

Slow-motion questioning exercise

What is it? An activity done with a large group of people.
Why would I use it? To emphasise the importance of thinking about and delivering powerful questions and getting feedback on those that were most helpful.
When would I use it? As a *'taster'* or *'starter'* session to give people a flavour of action learning.
How would I use it?

1. Working with a large group of people (around 20) who are interested in learning more about action learning, ask them to work in groups of about five or six people. Position chairs and tables so that everyone can see everyone else. Distribute blank filing cards to everyone.
2. Ask everyone in the large group to identify a *'knotty'* problem – a real issue which they currently face and on which they would value some help. This could be phrased as *'What is the most significant and important problem, issue or question facing me right now'.* Get them to write down their problem on one side of the card.
3. Get a volunteer from each group to describe and further elaborate their problem a little to the other small group members – a few minutes is normally enough – in order to give the group members some background. If the volunteer expresses the problem as a *'general'* issue, the facilitator may need to get them to take personal responsibility for it by asking them to rephrase it along the lines of *'How can I…?'* The other small group members turn their cards over, put their own issues out of their minds, listen carefully to the volunteer and do not interrupt.
4. Group members do not comment at this stage. Instead they listen and then write down a powerful question that they would like to ask the volunteer on the blank side of their card. Such a question should be one that they think might help that person to explore the particular issue with which they are concerned and to increase their understanding of the situation. Only questions are allowed – no comments.
5. In turn, each member of the small group asks their question. It is important that these really are questions – not advice giving or problem solving. The volunteer with the problem does not try to respond to these questions but instead listens and makes notes of each question, *'starring'* those that make them either wince or smile.
6. When each person has asked their question, the volunteer chooses the two or three questions which have had most impact on them and which they think will be most useful in finding a way forward – or which questions were most interesting or intriguing.
7. The volunteer then reads out those two or three questions and says exactly why they were important, challenging or intriguing. They might like to consider:
   a. Which questions they found most challenging or difficult
   b. Which questions they found most helpful
   c. Those questions that they feel that can answer now
   d. Those questions that feel that they cannot answer now
8. This provides useful feedback to the other group members on the relevance and utility of the questions which they posed. The volunteer may choose to attempt to answer them then and there – or they may not.

9. The larger group should then review the range and nature of the questions posed and whether they were, for example, open or closed, and what the major themes or angles emerging from them were. This can be expanded into a more general discussion on the quality of good questions.

SQIFED

What is it? A reflection model for use by set members.
Why would I use it? In order to encourage deeper reflection than what passes for normal in most situations.
When would I use it? After a set member has had had airtime, in order to deepen their reflection on the issue.
How would I use it? By encouraging the set member to ask:

S = What was my **s**ituation?
Q = What was the **q**uestion that I addressed?
I = What **i**nsightful questions were asked of me by set members?
F = What is now my **f**ocus of reflection?
E = What is the nature of my further **e**xploration of this?
D = What **d**evelopment pointers arise for me now? (1)

Thinking, feeling and willing exercise

What is it? An approach which focuses on the three major questions relevant to addressing an issue, problem or question. These questions are *'Who knows?'*, *'Who cares?'* and *'Who can?'* These questions correspond with the processes of thinking, feeling and willing.
Why would I use it? In order to avoid possible over-intellectualising approaches to problems by set members and instead to emphasise the equal importance of feeling and willing to that of thinking.
When would I use it? At a point when a large group of people is preparing to break down into action learning sets, as a means of highlighting the three major questions.
Alternatively, when set members seem to be *'stuck'* in using a purely rational (thinking) approach.
How would I use it?

Thinking is what takes place *'in the head'* – it is ideas, concepts, images, metaphors, theories and so on. Also, reflections, assumptions, judgements, mental models and frames of reference that lie behind the words and which cause us to see situations in particular lights.

Feeling relates to the emotions, sensations and energies that lie behind the words. Also atmosphere, ambience and vibrations.

Willing is concerned with wishes, purposes, intentions, power and energy which provides the drive, determination and effort needed to make things happen – the force that translates impulses and direction into practice.

The facilitator should split a large group into smaller groups of four people in each. One person talks for about 10–15 minutes about an issue that is important to them or about an aspect of their work that they have been thinking about recently. The remaining three people listen and do not interrupt or ask questions. They simply pay attention to what the first person is saying, one each of the three concentrating on:

- **Thinking:** What is being said by the first person, the thought patterns – is it logical? Detailed or general? Does it refer to the past, present or future? Who is being talked about and who is not? What images and metaphors are being used? What assumptions are being made?
- **Feeling:** What does the speaker seem to be feeling? Notice such things as gestures, posture, tone of voice, way of breathing, facial expressions and eye movements.
- **Willing:** What does the person want to do? What seems to be just a wish or a dream and what is a definite intention to act? The three listeners report back what they have each heard from the thinking, feeling and willing viewpoints to the first person, who needs to consider how what they report fits in with their own perceptions. This can then be repeated so that all four people have the same opportunity.

Trauma, trivia and joy

What is it? An exercise designed to deal with the natural anxiety of new set members, to allay their concerns and to help with the formation of the set.

Why would I use it? To help new set members to relax and to convey exactly how they are feeling with an informal immediacy.

When would I use it? At an initial set meeting.

How would I use it? Each person in the set is asked to describe briefly an event or incident, one of which could be described as a trauma, another as a trivia and a third as a joy, that has happened to them in the last few days. Each set member takes a turn at describing their events, including the facilitator, who may start and thus model the activity.

There is no discussion of the events. Other set members may convey their feelings and empathy with the occasional word, the effect of which is to create a warm and supportive atmosphere, to relax the set members and to help the set to get to know each other a little. Set members are asked not to invent events if they have not actually occurred. If a set member has just a joy and a trivia, then that is OK. If a set member wishes not to be included in this activity and to *'pass'* then that is also OK. Most set members, however, find the exercise quite light and certainly energising.

The exercise will take between 5 and 15 minutes, depending upon the numbers participating. It is important not to rush an individual set member but to convey the idea that this is a brief warm-up exercise to get the set going.

EXERCISES FOR ADDRESSING PROBLEMS IN THE WORKPLACE

Action planning

What is it? A list of the major and minor activities which have to be carried out in order to achieve an intended goal.

Why would I use it? Unless the actions which need to be taken are *'tied down'*, then there is a danger that an intended change will not happen, especially if it involves a number of people.

When would I use it? When planning how to put a change into action.

How would I use it? An effective action plan will be:

- ***Related*** to the broad aims or the desired future state of the change
- ***Specific***, with clearly defined activities
- ***Integrated***, with all parts of the action plan being connected
- ***Time-sequenced***, with a logical chronology of events
- ***Adaptable***, with contingency plans for possible unexpected events
- ***Realistic and achievable***

The process is to:

1. Generate all the ***major actions*** that need to be done. These might be *'layered'* from higher to lower organisational levels.
2. Identify any serious ***minor actions***, including those that may flow from the major actions, plus any ***links*** that need to be added in.
3. ***Sequence*** the major actions. What might proceed in tandem? What is dependent on earlier actions?
4. Insert the ***minor actions.***
5. A useful way of categorising major and minor actions is to divide them into:
   a. ***Quick wins*****:** Short-term, with low resource implications, but high impact. These can create energy and a momentum for change.
   b. ***Soft targets*****:** Short-term, with low resource implications, but lower impact. These should be tackled after quick wins.
   a. ***Challenging tasks*****:** Longer-term, with higher resource implications but with high impact. These are the actions which generally create the greatest change.
   b. ***Hold-offs*****:** Longer-term, with high resource implications and low impact. These are difficult challenges that should be left until other changes have been made or until circumstances change.
6. Devise sensible and realistic ***time scales*** for ongoing review, with ***milestone dates*** en route, and a date for final completion.
7. Identify the ***owners*** of each action, seeking equality of effort where possible.
8. The action plan should say ***who*** will do ***what*** and ***by when.***

Best boss exercise

What is it? A simple but effective process for identifying key work-based events when a major impact was made on a set member by someone who they considered to have been their *'best boss'*.
Why would I use it? In order to highlight the importance of support and challenge.
When would I use it? When a set member appears to be *'stuck'* in moving forward on an issue.
How would I use it? The facilitator should ask the set member to: Identify who their *'best boss'* actually was – or currently is.
Describe exactly what that person did to make such an impression on them.
Describe the impact which the behaviour of the *'best boss'* had on them.

It is likely that the actions of the *'best boss'* will have made an impact composed of some combination of support and challenge. The facilitator should then ask the set member *'What support and challenge do you need right now?'*

It is also possible to look at particularly difficult circumstances and pose the question *'What would my "best boss' do here?'* In this sense, we all carry around our *'best boss'* with us and can consult with him or her at any time.

Brainstorming

What is it? A process designed to produce a large number of ideas in a short period of time.
Why would I use it? To illustrate the multiplicity of potential ways forward and to highlight possible creative approaches.
When would I use it? As a means of generating possible ideas when a set member seems to have reached an impasse in a work situation.
How would I use it? The facilitator should explain the *'rules'* which are:

- ***Speak, then think***: The opposite of the usual advice
- ***Listen and build***: Upon what others contribute
- ***No 'Ah buts' are allowed***: Everything said goes on the list
- ***Leave it to brew***: After a break more ideas may occur

The set member describes the dilemma or dead-end which they seem to have reached and the facilitator asks for ideas from the other set members. Everything said is written down, usually on a flipchart, as the other set members express ideas quickly and spontaneously, more or less by free expression. No comments or criticism are permitted. Each set member is encouraged to say whatever they wish, no matter how unusual or unrealistic this may appear.

After a pause the facilitator asks the original set member to identify those ideas which have been generated which might well be feasible or actionable.

Circle of concern and circle of influence

What is it? A process to help a set member to discriminate between those issues over which they have no control and those which they can do something about.
Why would I use it? As a means of distinguishing between reactive and proactive behaviour in both the workplace and the set.
When would I use it? When a set member appears to be stuck in a reactive mode when addressing an issue.
How would I use it?

1. On a flipchart get a set member to draw a circle in which he/she depicts all the issues of concern related to the problem or issue with which they are dealing. The other set members contribute by probing and questioning, thereby identifying any other underlying concerns related to that issue.
2. The set member then transcribes onto a second flip chart two further circles discriminating between those issues that are in their circle of concern and those that are in their circle of influence. The larger circle is the circle of concern and placed within it is the circle of influence. A way of determining into which circle the issues are placed is by listening to the language used and distinguishing between the ***'have's*** (circle of concern) and the ***'be's*** (circle of influence). For example:

'Have's' (Reactive)	'Be's' (Proactive)
'I'll only be happy when I'm fully staffed'	*'I can be a better role model'*
'If only I had a boss who wasn't...'	*'I can be more organised...'*
'If I had respect from..'	*'I can be more understanding...'*
'If I had a degree...'	*'I will be more diligent...'*
'If only the setting was better..'	*'I can approach them directly..'*

The nature of the reactive approach is an absolving of responsibility and a "*them and us*" reading of reality. The nature of the proactive approach is an inside-out focus, being value-driven and a recognition that change starts with the individual.

3. Once visually displayed on the flipcharts, an exploration can then take place of the steps that are needed in order to behave more proactively.

Concept analysis

What is it? A tool to understand an issue and to explore it in more detail by clarifying it so that it can be studied in much greater depth, as a means to focus efforts in a more organised way.
Why would I use it? In order to gain clarity about a concept, issue or situation.
When would I use it? At an early stage of a set member working on a particular issue.
How would I use it? Concept analysis uses a three-way approach to exploring the:

- ***Antecedents***: What needs to be in place in order to make something happen.
- ***Attributes***: What the characteristics are of a particular change.
- ***Consequences***: What the positive and negative outcomes of such a change would be.

The set can be broken up into twos or threes in order to brainstorm each element of concept analysis and then to feed back to the whole set. Alternatively, the entire set may do this work. The discussion should contribute to the actions necessary to take the issue forward.

Dealing with anger in others

What is it? A series of techniques for dealing with angry colleagues.
Why would I use it? In order to reduce anger levels and to promote listening, empathy and effective communication.
When would I use it? When a set member reported regular occasions when they encountered anger in their dealings with work colleagues in their own or other organisations.
How would I use it? There are five key activities which can help to deal with anger in others. They are:

1. ***Keep calm***: The set member needs to make sure that they do not panic or lose their own temper. This is obviously easy to say but not always easy to do. If they do lose self-control then they are less likely to dissipate the other person's anger in order to move on to addressing the issue.
2. ***Listen***: The set member needs to pay full attention to the angry person so that they can gather as many facts as possible as well as identifying any other underlying feelings that may have generated the anger.

3. ***Empathise***: The set member needs to make sure that they communicate their understanding of the other person's views and feelings. They should agree with what they can honestly agree with, including admitting the possibility that they might be part of the problem. Some typical responses that can be used to show empathy are:
   a. *'Yes, I can see how angry you are.'*
   b. *'I can understand that you feel that way.'*
   c. *'What exactly did she say?'*
   d. *'It has been going on for quite a long time, hasn't it.'*
   e. *'Yes, I didn't get it finished by the due date as I had hoped.'*
   f. *'Maybe I didn't really give enough thought to that possibility.'*
   g. *'I'm glad you're telling me about this.'*
   h. *'I want to try to resolve this with you.'*
4. ***Don't argue***: Until the anger and any other emotions are out of the way, there is no point at all in trying to use logical, rational argument. It is only likely to fuel the anger. Once the anger is dissipated the set member needs to try to move on to resolution of the issue, with phrases such as *'OK, now let's see what we can do to sort this out between us.'*
5. ***Save face***: This needs to be done throughout the discussion by:
   a. The set member agreeing with what they can
   b. Focusing on the issue and not the personality
   c. Using the word *'I'* instead of *'you'*

This serves to respect the set member's rights while at the same time not violating the rights of others. The need to save face can be particularly strong once the chemistry of anger has dissipated. Many people experience remorse in hindsight. They then feel guilty about their loss of self-control or foolish for having lost their temper or the extent to which they have gone *'over the top'*. So the set member should use reflective, non-judgemental and empathic statements such as:

- *'Yes, you did go a bit over the top, but I can well understand why.'*
- *'We all get angry at times and it helps to get the emotion out of the way so we can then tackle the issue together.'*

The set member needs to make sure that they accurately reflect the feelings the other person is expressing and that what they say is honest and in no way patronising.

Dealing with face-to-face criticism

What is it? A series of tips for set members who are faced with face-to-face criticism when pursuing their issue of choice.

Why would I use it? To help a set member consider a variety of strategies for dealing with face-to-face criticism.

When would I use it? When a set member has been non-plussed by receiving unexpected criticism directly.

How would I use it? Offer the tips in handout form and use them as the basis for a one-to-one dialogue with the set member.

1. ***Expect to feel defensive***: It is quite normal to feel defensive when we are criticised – our brains perceive criticism as a threat (to our self-esteem, our self-respect and so on) and

consequently we often go into a version of the *'fight or flight'* response which is the way in which we protect ourselves in what we experience as threatening situations. Fight/flight feelings may be experienced as embarrassment, humiliation or anger.

2. ***Don't let your feelings dictate your response*:** Notice your feelings and recognise them for what they are – a normal human response to a perceived threat. Feeling embarrassed, for example, does not mean that the other person's criticism is justified; feeling angry does not mean the other person is wrong. The trick when handling criticism is to go into *'head'* mode rather than *'feelings'* mode. This means acting in a coolly professional manner even though you may be feeling anxious or irritated. Try and view the issue as a problem to be solved rather than a debate which you have to win. This is easy to say, but harder to do – it takes both commitment and practice.
3. ***Listen carefully*:** Let the other person say what they have to say. Use good active listening behaviours (nodding, saying *'uh huh'*, and so on) in order to show that you are taking their criticism on board. While you are listening you can also use the time to collect yourself. Letting the other person have their say also prevents the temperature of the conversation from rising (which is exactly what happens when we interrupt the other person before they have finished).
4. ***Ask some questions*:** This will:
   a. Give you more information on what it is that the other person is unhappy about.
   b. Show the other person that you are prepared to discuss the matter in a mature and rational way.
5. ***Make sure your questions are neutral*:** It's tempting to use a question to try and score a point (*'Are you seriously accusing me of ...?'*) but point-scoring usually leads to conflict. Examples of neutral questions are *'Could you say a bit more about that?'* and *'Have you noticed this on more than one occasion?'* – but be careful not to sound like a lawyer cross-examining a witness!
6. ***Respond*:** Once you have listened and asked questions, you are left with one of two responses – to either agree or disagree. By using this Listen/Ask Questions approach you can accept criticism but still walk away from the conversation pleased with how you conducted yourself. If you disagree with the other person, you have at least shown them that you have taken on board their concerns, rather than reacting out of an instinctive need to defend yourself.
7. ***Ask for time*:** If you are taken aback by the criticism and are having difficulty in controlling your emotions, then you might suggest to the other person that you talk through the issue at some other time. If you do this, then it is important that you do follow-through and arrange such a meeting.

Drama triangle

What is it? A psychological and social model of human interaction derived from transactional analysis.

Why would I use it? In order to encourage a set member to look beyond purely rational explanations of what is happening when they seem to be *'stuck'*. It describes a mind game – an unconscious game played by innocent people.

When would I use it? When a set member describes a continuing situation where they portray themselves as a Victim or possibly a Rescuer. As an explanatory device, the Drama Triangle can cast light on what is happening in such a triangular relationship.

How would I use it? The model offers three habitual psychological roles which people take in a situation. They are:

***Victim*:** The person who is habitually pressurised, coerced or persecuted.
***Persecutor*:** The person who pressures, coerces or persecutes the Victim.
***Rescuer*:** The person who intervenes in this interaction, seemingly out of a desire to help the situation or the underdog. The Rescuer has a mixed or covert motive so that they can benefit egotistically from being the one who rescues. They have a surface motive of solving the problem, and appear to make great efforts to solve it, but also have a hidden motive not to succeed, or to succeed in a way from which they benefit.

The relationship between the Victim and the Rescuer can be one of co-dependency –the Rescuer keeps the Victim dependent on them by playing into their victimhood. The Victim gets their needs met by having the Rescuer take care of them.

Force field analysis

What is it? A means of gathering information about what might drive improvement and to balance this with the opposing forces that might be barriers to change.
Why would I use it? Any problem can be considered as a dynamic balance of forces working in opposite directions. Forces working in one direction (helping forces) are opposed by forces working in the opposite direction (hindering forces). No change will take place unless an imbalance in these forces is created.
When would I use it? Early on in considering a project or change issue. As the project progresses it can also be reviewed regularly using this tool. It can be done by individuals or by groups.
How would I use it?

1. The problem should be summarised and defined in an explicit fashion, with no use of bullet points, usually as *'How can we...?'*
2. A description of a better or improved or desirable situation should also be written along similar lines.
3. Ideas are generated to create lists of all the present helping and hindering forces, with the helping forces pressing towards the improved situation and the hindering forces pushing against change.
4. Each item on both lists is given a score from 1 to 10 in terms of how easy it would be to change - 10 is easiest, 1 is hardest.
5. Do the calculations – the highest scores are the easiest to deal with, the lowest are those that you may have to work around, rather than on.
6. Generate strategies to deal with the problem and move towards the desired state. This could involve:
   a. Changing the strength of a force
   b. Changing the direction of a force
   c. Withdrawing hindering forces
   d. Adding new helping forces

It is often best to begin by working on hindering forces because increasing the helping forces often simultaneously creates resistance.

Perceptual positioning

What is it? A technique whereby a set member can mentally review (or preview) a situation from a number of different standpoints in order to enrich their appreciation of what is involved.

Why would I use it? The approach:

1. Improves understanding of other people
2. Enables the set member to think more flexibly and creatively
3. Provides an opportunity to stand back and to consider issues dispassionately
4. Helps the set member to appreciate the influence of their verbal and non-verbal behaviour on others, and the influence of their behaviour on them.

When would I use it? When the set member needs to review an interaction with another person, or to prepare for a forthcoming one.

How would I use it? The approach uses two *'rounds'*. The first round provides insights into the current situation, while the second round enables the set member to benefit from the insights gained in the first round, while mentally *'wiring-in'* the learning.

Round 1:

- ***First perspective*:** The set member sees the situation through their own eyes, running through the meeting or interaction as if they are actually in it. Attention needs to be paid to personal thoughts, feelings and needs.
- ***Second perspective*:** The set member has to imagine what it is like to be the other person – to put themselves in their shoes and to look back at themselves, seeing, hearing and feeling as the other person. How is that *'you over there'* coming across? Are they in rapport or not? Are they exhibiting respect? Are they taking the other person's views into account?
- ***Third perspective*:** Here the set member needs to take a detached viewpoint and imagine that they are looking at themselves and the other person *'over there'* – seeing the two of them speaking, gesturing, etc. Particular attention needs to be paid to non-verbal behaviour such as the body language and the tone of their voices. The set member needs to consider, as a result of taking this view, what advice they would wish to give to themselves about how they are handling the situation.

***Round 2*:**

The process is repeated using the insights and advice from Round 1, with the set member running through it with the new behaviours – firstly as themselves, then as the other person and finally the detached view. The set member should then be encouraged to think of upcoming events in which these insights may be useful.

Preparing a business case

What is it? A means of making a case for a desired change to the organisation or organisations in both financial and non-financial terms.

Why would I use it? When making the case for a proposed change to the wider organisation or organisations.

When would I use it? When the processes of diagnosis and analysis are complete and the desired way forward is clear, but the wider organisation or organisations need to be convinced.

How would I use it? There are six headings usually expected in a business case, although some organisations may have developed their own model. The general template is:

1. ***Proposition or summary*:** A two- or three-sentence summary of the change that is being proposed.
2. ***Context*:** Two or three sentences about why the proposed change really matters to health, social or community care and to the organisation or organisations concerned.
3. ***Scale of change*:** Say whether the proposed change involves a small or larger part of the organisation or organisations. Also to say whether any new roles are involved and how many there may possibly be.
4. ***Financial analysis*:** This includes:
   Estimated costs, split between:
   a. ***Non-recurring (or one-off) costs*:** such as project management, equipment, recruitment, initial training, evaluation, changes to accommodation, pump priming, and so on.
   b. ***Recurring (or continuing) costs*:** salaries, wages, payments.
   ***Estimated savings*:** These are more difficult to identify than costs, but remember that a business case involves looking at ways of doing things differently, not simply ways of using extra staff. Look at what the organisation or organisations may be currently spending, which is often very different from what is budgeted for, and look at what could potentially be saved over time. Look for the savings in staff costs such as a reduced use of agency and locum staff, reduced staff turnover and from reduced multiple visits by patients to hospital, less complaints and less paperwork, for example.
   ***Timing*:** An analysis of costs and savings over the relevant financial years.
5. ***Non-financial impact*:** Even if the main reason for a change is an improvement in quality, it is probably important in these times to quantify it as much as can be achieved, especially if there is a cost associated with the change. Try to quantify the likely impact of the change on key performance targets.
6. ***Evidence and risk*:** Say why you believe the proposed change will work. Give examples of small-scale pilots or a history of success elsewhere. Include examples of the potential risks and how you might plan to prevent them.

Role negotiation

What is it? A technique directed at the work relationships between members of a team. As an approach it avoids probing into the personal likes and dislikes of team members or their personal feelings about each other. It is a structure for controlled negotiations between people in which each person agrees in writing to change certain work behaviours in exchange for changes in behaviour by another person.

Why would I use it? In order for set members to negotiate changes in the behaviour of their work colleagues in exchange for changes in their own.

When would I use it? Where set members experienced unrealistic demands on them by their work colleagues and are prepared to negotiate towards a solution.

How would I use it? The focus is on work behaviours, not on feelings about people. There is a need for a set member to be quite specific in stating what it is that they would like to be changed. All expectations or demands must be written down. No-one agrees to change any particular behaviours unless there is a quid pro quo in which the other person must also agree to a change. Individuals negotiate with each other to arrive at a *'contract'* of what behaviours each will change.

1. ***Individual work:*** Individuals should reflect upon significant and recent (i.e. within the last year) work-based incidents involving each of their colleagues in turn, in which they feel they were particularly effective or ineffective. Questions to consider might be:
   a. What happened – and what didn't happen?
   b. What else might have happened?
   Based upon reflection on these incidents, there is a need to be quite specific and to write down for each person what, in order to be more effective in your work role, you need them to:

   Keep on doing (or do better): Because you appreciate, value and welcome it and because it is helping you in your own job performance.

   Do more of (or do better): Because you need an increase in these behaviours in order to perform well or to perform better.

   Do less of (or stop doing): Because it causes you problems and creates obstacles to your more effective performance.

   Keep to an upper limit of three behaviours under each of the headings.
2. ***Negotiating pairs:*** Work in pairs with each colleague in turn to discuss the most important behaviour changes that you want from them and the changes that you are willing to make yourself. A quid pro quo is needed at this stage – each person must give something in order to get something, along the lines of *'If you do X, I'll do Y'.* Negotiation is complete when both individuals are satisfied that they will receive a reasonable return on whatever it is that they are agreeing to give. The *'contract'* should be written-up, with each person having a copy and a review date should be agreed to determine whether the *'contracts'* have been honoured and to assess the impact on both individual and team effectiveness.

Role set analysis

What is it? A means of helping a set member to analyse and think through what is expected of them and how these expectations may possibly conflict and so cause problems.

Why would I use it? To help the set member to understand that some of the expectations laid on them may be contradictory and unrealistic. Analysing such conflicting demands is a first step to managing them or changing them.

When would I use it? When a set member describes a situation where they are faced with two or more sets of expectations which contradict each other and are unclear about which to meet and why.

How would I use it?

1. Ask the set member to draw themselves at the centre of a sheet of paper with, around them, the key individuals and groups that they have to interact with in order to do their daily job.
2. Ask the set member to write down beside each identified person or group what they believe that person or group wants, needs or expects of them, and conversely, what they want, need or expect of that person or group.
3. It is likely that this process will indicate areas where there is conflict – for example, between what people expect and what they get, or between what is wanted and what can be provided.

Say what you see

What is it? A method to use when things are not going well for a set member and when they are confused as to what to do about it. Such situations might include:

- A failure of communications between the set member and her staff – she keeps asking for something to happen and it doesn't happen.
- Something not working between the set member and another person.
- A team or group not behaving how the set member believes it should – for example, missing deadlines, not taking responsibility or not being constructive in meetings.
- Things going wrong repeatedly – despite promises to fix them.

In all these cases, it is possible to see the problem but not know how to fix it.

Why would I use it? In situations of ambiguity where the way forward seems clear to the set member but not to colleagues and staff.

When would I use it? By the set member in a meeting with colleagues and staff.

How would I use it? It comprises a simple four-stage model:

1. **Say what you see:** For example, the set member might say to colleagues and staff '*I notice that we keep returning to the same issue without moving forward*' or '*I notice that there are a lot of raised voices*' or '*I notice that people are looking out of the window a lot*' or '*I notice that half the group have not come to the meeting*' or '*I notice that we have not actually implemented the decisions that we made two months ago*'.
2. **Check for agreement:** This is vital. Does the individual or group see things your way? If they do not, then it is your problem. If they do, then it is a shared problem. If it is shared, then you can go on to the next step.
3. **Ask for suggestions:** Ask '*What do you think we should do about this*?' Notice the 'we', not 'you' or 'I'.
4. **Wait:** This is the most important and hardest part. Our own anxiety often drives us to fill the vacuum of silence but leaving the time and space for a response is crucial. If a response is not forthcoming it is possible to start again at the first stage by saying, 'I notice that I'm not getting an answer. Is this how you see it?'

Six action shoes

What is it? A tool to help to decide exactly what kind of action to take on an issue.

Why would I use it? To help a set member to decide on what is the best way forward in taking practical action on an issue.

When would I use it? As a set member begins to move from a diagnostic towards an action phase of their work.

How would I use it? Shoes imply action – they are means of reaching a destination. Each pair of action shoes is assigned a different colour and covers one particular action or style of approach. Action is considered as a two-step process:

1. Ask 'What type of action is required here?'
2. Put on the appropriate action shoes and behave in that style. The shoes are:

***Orange gumboots*:** To put on in order to take urgent action to overcome a crisis or to deal with an emergency situation.

***Pink slippers*:** To put on in order to take caring or helping action in a situation where it is vital to consider and to respect human feelings.

***Navy formal shoes*:** To put on in order to take action which requires authority or rules and regulations to be established or adhered to. When action should follow set routines.

***Brown sensible shoes*:** To put on in order to take practical action – that which seems sensible in the situation.

***Purple riding boots*:** To put on in order to take *'extraordinary'* action that is defined by the wearer of the shoes.

***Grey sneakers*:** To put on in order to investigate and collect information.

Six thinking hats

What is it? A means to plan thinking processes in a detailed and cohesive way and, in doing so, to think more effectively.

Why would I use it? To help set members to unscramble their thinking so that a thinker can use one thinking mode (or hat) at a time, instead of trying to do everything at once. It helps the set member to think logically and to explore different areas one at a time. It can also validate emotional aspects of an issue which are acknowledged and placed alongside facts and logic. This is important where there is a lot of emotion attached to an issue which colours all other thinking.

When would I use it? When set members cannot think straight about a situation and their thoughts are jumbled up.

How would I use it? There are six imaginary hats, each a different colour. At any moment a thinker may choose to put on one of the hats or may be asked to put on or take off a hat. The hats are:

***Black hat*:** Specifically concerned with negative assessment. The black hat thinker points out what is wrong, incorrect or in error. This hat gives people permission to talk about *'gripes and groans'* and gets them out of the way.

***White hat*:** This hat indicates neutrality and is used to collect or identify facts and figures. It does not offer interpretations or opinions.

***Red hat*:** The red hat legitimises emotions and feelings as an important part of thinking. When using this hat there should never be any attempt to justify the feelings or to provide a logical basis for them.

***Yellow hat*:** This hat is about positive thinking and being constructive. It symbolises sunshine, brightness and optimism and is concerned with positive assessment, just as the black hat is concerned with negative assessment.

***Green hat*:** The green hat is for creative thinking and symbolises fertility, growth and the value of seeds. It implies that there is a need to go beyond the known and obvious.

***Blue hat*:** This is the *'control'* hat which is responsible for summaries, overviews and conclusions.

Strategies, strengths, resources, insights review

What is it? An approach which helps people to review the strategies that they have found useful, the strengths they have drawn upon, the resources they have discovered and the insights that have made a difference to them – in order to identify their personal *'toolkit'*.

Why would I use it? To encourage set members to take stock of the approaches which they already use well – what works for them – as a baseline for further development.

When would I use it? When a set member appears to be overcome with self-doubt and apprehension concerning their self-worth and their ability to effect change.

How would I use it? The approach can be done on a personal basis, but sometimes a fellow set member or work colleague can be invited to do it, as sometimes others have a clearer picture of how we are than we do ourselves. The process is to remember a challenging time in the past which you found a way through. Think back to what helped to find the way through by looking at the following areas:

***Strategies*:** What were the personal strategies that were used? Asking for help? Using problem-solving approaches?

***Strengths*:** What were the strengths drawn upon in order to get through that challenging time? Courage? Foresight? Determination? A sense of humour? Flexibility? Ability to communicate?

***Resources*:** What were the resources mobilised for personal nourishment, inspiration, guidance or support? Family? Friends? Colleagues? Mentors? Support groups? Places where a sense of safety and calm prevails?

***Insights*:** Ideas, perspectives or sayings that were previously found useful. For example, the saying *'I can't, but we can'* or the insight that personal and group resilience are powerfully intertwined.

SWOT analysis

What is it? A tool for analysing the strengths, weaknesses, opportunities and threats facing an organisation, team or individual and using the results to identify priorities for action.

Why would I use it? Internal and external factors need to be considered simultaneously when identifying those aspects of an organisation or team that needs to be changed. Strengths and weaknesses are typically internal to the organisation or team, while opportunities and threats are usually external.

When would I use it? When considering a statement of purpose for an organisation or team.

How would I use it? Work with a group to identify:

***Strengths*:** The things which we are good at. What is it that we have going for us?

***Weaknesses*:** The things which we are poor at. The mistakes which we keep making. The downside of the organisation or team.

***Opportunities*:** Things that are happening or that are anticipated to happen that might help us. New developments coming over the horizon that we can capitalise on.

***Threats*:** New things coming up that look bad for us. The problems lurking around the next corner.

The next phase, which involves identifying priorities for future action involves:

For ***Strengths*:** *How can we maximise and extend them?*
For ***Weaknesses*:** *How can we minimise or overcome them?*
For ***Opportunities*:** *How can we best exploit them?*
For ***Threats*:** *How can we avoid or counter them?*

The change equation

What is it? A tool which helps to scope-out a range of relevant factors in bringing about change.
Why would I use it? Early consideration of resistance to change and the causes of such resistance can be helpful in deciding on necessary actions.
When would I use it? At the commencement of a project or planned change.
How would I use it? The change equation shows that we need to recognise and understand the many factors involved in a change in order to overcome anticipated resistance. It is expressed in terms of an algebraic formula:

Let **A** = The individual, group or organisation's ***level of dissatisfaction with the present situation*** and the pressure for change which this engenders. Questions to ask here are:

How satisfied are people with the current state of things?
Is any of this dissatisfaction shared with colleagues?
How is the dissatisfaction understood and experienced?

Let **B** = ***A clear and shared vision of a better future*** – how things could potentially be and what the changed situation would look like. Questions to consider here are:

What do people really want for themselves, their colleagues and the patients/clients/ service users and the populations and communities which they serve?
What are their values and beliefs, goals and desires?
What could the new change look like?

Let **C** = The ***capacity of the individual, group or organisation to change*** in terms of competence, skills, orientation, resources, etc. Important questions here are:

What resources are needed in order to achieve the change, including capability and energy?
How can these resources be acquired, generated or shared?
Have people shown in the past that they are willing to try out new ideas?
Can you identify those people who are personally and professionally respected and who have demonstrated energy and capability to make changes and put them in contact with others?

Let **D** = ***Acceptable and do-able first steps*** – what can be done immediately to kick-start matters in order to make the change happen? The key question is:

What first steps could people undertake which everyone could agree would be a movement in the right direction?

Let **R** = ***Resistance*** – the assumed cost to the individual, group or organisation of making the change, in terms of finance, time, effort or '*hassle*'.

So the change equation is that change will be resisted unless:

$$\mathbf{A \times B \times C \times D} \text{ is greater than } \mathbf{R}$$

If the product of these four factors (**A, B, C** and **D**) is greater than **R**, then change is possible, because of a multiplier effect. If, however, any one of these factors is absent or low then the product will be low and therefore not capable of overcoming the resistance. When any of the four factors are missing there are predictable results:

Where **B** × **C** × **D** exists, but **A** is missing or low, it means that the change issue will *'go to the bottom of the in-tray'* and the urgent will drive out the important.
Where **A** × **C** × **D** exists, but **B** is missing or low then, after a fast and furious start-up, the change will simply run down or fade out.
Where **A** × **B** × **D** exists, but **C** is missing or low then, in the absence of capacity to manage change successfully, anxiety and frustration will result.
Where **A** × **B** × **C** exists, but **D** is missing or low, the change effort will be haphazard and there will be a succession of re-launches and *'false-starts'*.

It can be helpful to look back at previous change activities using this approach to ask what might have gone wrong – in order to plan the new project or change more carefully.

The five 'whys'

What is it? A tool which helps to identify the root causes of a problem, rather than the symptoms or *'presenting'* issues.
Why would I use it? To provide a number of different perspectives on the same issue or problem, providing a broad base from which to consider options for action.
When would I use it? When wishing to delve deeper into the underlying causes of a problem as a means of identifying the basic factors.
How would I use it?

1. Working with a group or individually, the problem or issue should be clearly defined.
2. Ask yourself or the group *'Why?'* and note down all the answers generated.
3. For each response to the *'Why?'* question, again ask *'Why?'* and so on until the group or yourself can offer no further answers.
4. In total, ask *'Why?'* five times to get to the root causes of the problem or issue.
5. Use the answers to generate an action plan.

Working on 'trigger' events

What is it? A means of identifying, decoding and experimenting with *'trigger'* events which cause a set member to experience a major upset.
Why would I use it? To encourage a set member to examine specific events which triggered negative feelings in them and to decide on practical ways forward.
When would I use it? When a set member describes regularly occurring situations which generate negative emotions, but cannot see a way to deal with them.
How would I use it?

1. Ask the set member to think of a recent time when they felt relatively upset. Do they know exactly what triggered it? How long did they *'stay under'*? What brought them out of it?
2. Ask the set member to consider the event that triggered their upset. Did the event leave them with a *'can't do'*, *'can't say'* or *'can't get my needs met'* feeling? Ask them to try not to focus on what *'they'* did in the event – the most important thing is for the set member to work out how it affected them.

3. Depending upon what the set member's *'can't'* is, ask them to consider the following questions:
   a. How might you do the thing you want to do anyway?
   b. How could you find a way to say what you need to say?
   c. How might you find a different way to get your needs met?
4. If the set member still has a *'can't'* ask them to work with another set member or a colleague at work to help to find a personal strategy to make it a *'can'*.

Z technique

What is it? A process composed of questions based on the framework of the Myers-Briggs Type Instrument (MBTI).
Why would I use it? To help to widen the focus in seeking to address a problem.
When would I use it? When set members have become bogged-down or are trying to address a problem by concentrating only on a particular aspect.
How would I use it? A set member is invited to answer four questions in relation to the question or issue which they are trying to resolve.

1. What are the facts? (Sensing)
2. What are the possibilities? If we had no constraints, what would be possible?
3. (Intuition)
4. What are the logical implications of any choices I might make? (Thinking)
5. What is the likely impact on other people of any of my choices? (Feeling)

EXERCISES FOR REVIEWING SET PROCESSES

Action learning problem brief

What is it? A simple set of questions which will help you to think through a suitable problem, opportunity or issue for working on through action learning.
Why would I use it? To ensure that, prior to attending the first action learning set meeting, you had carefully thought through the problem situation which you are addressing.
When would I use it? Before the first action learning set meeting.
How would I use it? By considering the following questions:

1. Describe your problem, challenge or situation in a single sentence.
2. Why is this important:
   a. To you?
   b. To your organisation?
3. What have you already tried that hasn't worked so far?
4. How will you recognise progress on this problem?
5. Who else would like to see progress on this problem?
6. What difficulties do you anticipate?
7. What are the benefits if this problem is reduced or resolved?
   a. To me?
   b. To other people?
   c. To the organisation or organisations?

Action learning set 'contract'

What is it? A statement of the relative responsibilities of the key stakeholders associated with an action learning set.
Why would I use it? To ensure that there is a clarity of expectations between all the major players.
When would I use it? Prior to, or shortly after, the first meeting of an action learning set.
How would I use it? The *'contract'* sets out the responsibilities of the individuals concerned so that there can be no confusion or ambiguity over who is responsible for what. What is shown here should be regarded only as a template, which may be modified or added-to in order to suit local circumstances.

Set member:

- To work with the sponsor in order to identify and agree on an appropriate issue or issues which will be worked on at and between set meetings, accepting that the issue chosen may evolve or change as the set progresses.
- To attend regularly all set meetings and to support and challenge fellow set members as they work on their issues and challenges.
- To listen attentively to other set members, and to be open and generous with suggestions and constructive ideas.
- To follow-up action agreed at the set meeting back in the workplace and to report on progress at future set meetings.
- To respect confidentiality and individual differences and to be open in learning through action.
- To take part in evaluation activity.

Sponsor:

- To identify carefully those individuals for whom participation in an action learning set would be a useful development activity, from the point of view of both that individual and the organisation or organisations.
- To become as well-informed about the purpose and process of action learning in general, and of the work of the sponsored set member in particular, in order to make informed decisions and choices.
- To work with the set member in order to identify appropriate issues which will be worked on in the set, accepting that these may evolve or change as the set develops.
- To support the regular attendance of the set member at set meetings by accepting that set activity is a worthwhile and valuable use of time and an investment for the future for that individual and for the organisation.
- To help the set member with the implementation of actions in the workplace that emerge from the set meetings.
- To take part in evaluation activity.

Facilitator:

- To model appropriate behaviour for the set membership, such as high-quality listening skills and the asking of useful questions.
- To be active in the early life of the set in order to foster a sense of collective identity and mutual interdependence amongst the set members.

- Thereafter, to be timely and appropriate in interventions in the set's life, concentrating largely on the process (how set members and the set as a whole are working) – with the aim of enabling individual and group learning to take place.
- To encourage set members to focus on agreed actions.
- To take part in evaluation activity.

Action/reflection map

What is it? A simple process to help set members to get the balance between action and reflection in the work of the set *'right'* for them. It also shows how that balance may differ for different set members.

Why would I use it? In order to reveal that the requisite balance between action and reflection will vary between different set members, so that more or less reflection or action may be engendered for each person.

When would I use it? As part of the review at the end of a set meeting.

How would I use it? Each set member is asked to say how they felt the emphasis had been on taking action in the workplace during the set meeting on a scale of 0 (No emphasis) to 10 (Complete emphasis). Then they are asked to say how they felt the emphasis had been on reflection and review during the set meeting on a similar scale of 0 (No emphasis) to 10 (Complete emphasis).

The scores for each set member are then plotted onto a simple flip chart or wallchart graph with two axes – one for Action and the other for Reflection, ranging from 0 to 10 on each axis. This shows how individual set members experienced the set meeting and can stimulate discussion about the appropriate degree of emphasis on action and reflection needed in future set meetings.

Appreciative introductions

What is it? A simple process for introducing set members to each other and to start fostering a positive mood or climate within the newly formed set.

Why would I use it? At the outset, and especially when set members have never previously experienced action learning, there will be a degree of anxiety and apprehension concerning the first meeting with a group of *'strangers'*. This will establish a positive beginning to the set's working, as well as effecting introductions for each set member.

When would I use it? At the first set meeting.

How would I use it? Set members are asked to pair up and to share with each other answers to such questions as:

Things I appreciate about working in my organisation.
Things I appreciate about working on or addressing this problem.
Things I appreciate about being part of this group.
Things I appreciate about myself.

Each partner has about 12 minutes to explore these – so around 25 minutes in total for this phase of the exercise.

Each individual in turn introduces their partner to the whole set, reporting what the partner said in response to the questions, and with the introduced adding:

What I appreciate about the conversation we have just had is ...

Learning log

What is it? A tool which can help to structure report-backs to a set meeting on the actions taken in the workplace and the challenges met.

Why would I use it? To ensure that the workplace activities are reviewed and considered in preparation for explaining these to the other set members.

When would I use it? Prior to attending a set meeting, in order to get thoughts in order.

How would I use it? The learning log simply involves responding to the following questions:

1. What was it I planned to do after the last set meeting?
2. How did I go about it? What actions did I take?
3. What were the responses to those actions?
4. What were the outcomes or consequences?
5. Was it what I anticipated?
   a. If Yes, what went well?
   b. If No, what could I have done or said differently?
   c. My reflections on what happened.
6. What was I thinking?
7. What was I feeling? Did my feelings match my actions?
8. Did I do or say what I'd planned to do or say?
   a. If not, what was stopping me?
   b. What did I choose not to say or do and why did I make that choice?
9. What have I learned?
10. What do I want to focus on next time or in the future?

Set meeting review worksheet

What is it? An aid to reviewing the set meeting, capturing the learning derived and emphasising the importance of follow-up action in the workplace.

Why would I use it? In order to give some shape to the set meeting review process, balancing individual insights with the need for progress back at work.

When would I use it? At the close of a set meeting.

How would I use it? At the close of a set meeting all set members spend about five minutes reflecting individually and privately on the work of the set before sharing their results with fellow set members.

My problem/issue/opportunity: The three key things I have learned about my problem/issue opportunity today are:

1.
2.
3.

Myself**:** The one thing I've learned about myself today is:

Action**:** My action steps before the next meeting are:

1.
2.
3.

Other set members: The most interesting things I've learned today about the problems/issues/opportunities facing each of the other set members are:

1.
2.
3.
4.
5.
6.

Support/challenge map

What is it? A simple process to help set members get the balance between support and challenge in the work of the set *'right'* for them. It also shows how that balance may differ for different set members.

Why would I use it? In order to reveal that the balance between support and challenge will vary between different set members, so that more or less challenge or support may be engendered for each person.

When would I use it? As part of the review at the end of a set meeting.

How would I use it? Each set member is asked to say how they felt they had been supported in the set meeting on a scale of 0 (Not supported) to 10 (Totally supported). Then they are asked to say how they felt they had been challenged in the set meeting on a similar scale of 0 (Not challenged) to 10 (Fully challenged). The scores for each set member are then plotted onto a simple flip chart or wallchart graph with two axes – one for Support and the other for Challenge, ranging from 0 to 10 on each axis. This shows how individual set members experienced the set meeting and can stimulate discussion about the appropriate degree of support and challenge needed in future set meetings.

ACTION LEARNING ORGANISATIONS

A number of organisations, associations and other bodies exist in order to promote and support the use and further development of action learning. They include:

Action Learning: Research & Practice

This is essentially the major *'house journal'* for action learning. It aims to publish articles that advance knowledge and assist the development of practice through the processes of action learning. The articles which it publishes aim to create empirically grounded theory which widens the understanding of action and learning in professional and organisational settings. The purpose of the published papers is to encourage action learning practitioners to gain new insights into their work and to help them to improve their effectiveness and contribution to their clients and to the wider community. Because action learning promotes the creative integration of thinking and doing, theory and practice, academic and practitioner, all contributors are asked to strive to hold these often-diverse perspectives together. Articles which cross the conventional boundaries of professions, organisations and communities are particularly welcome.

There are three types of contribution:

- ***Refereed papers*:** These are articles which seek to generate new insights and theory which illuminate the idea of action learning.
- ***Accounts of practice*:** These are articles which express the concept of action learning by presenting examples of, and explaining how, action learning has led to the development of new perspectives and new ideas and how the practitioner has changed practice because of insights gained through collaborative learning.
- ***Reviews*:** These include review articles, surveys of fields of practice, conference reports and book reviews of relevant publications.

For further information, go to: www.tandfonline.com/toc/CALR20/current#.VM9iEGisWT8 or contact the editorial department at Taylor & Francis Group:

Taylor & Francis
4 Park Square
Milton Park
ABINGDON
Oxon
OX14 4RN
UK

The journal also organises an international action learning conference which takes place every two years.

International Foundation for Action Learning (IFAL): UK chapter

Originally created in 1977 as the Action Learning Trust. IFAL UK is a key source of information and support for those who practice and those who are simply interested in knowing more about action learning.

IFAL's core values are:

- ***Passion*:** Deep feelings about action learning and the powerful effects it can have on individuals, teams and organisations.
- ***Knowledge*:** To learn and contribute to the body of knowledge around action learning; to be open to new experiences, ideas and opinions to raise the standard of practice.
- ***Service*:** To be helpful to others in supporting their growth and development; to make a difference and to keep the debate about action learning alive, current and relevant.

The use of action learning is encouraged by:

- ***Providing information*:** Responding to requests and promoting discussion by phone and letter and via the IFAL group at LinkedIn.
- ***Library*:** IFAL has over 1000 items of writing about action learning, many of which are not available elsewhere.
- ***IFAL e-letter*:** A regular e-letter provides the opportunity for members to share their ideas and experiences and spread news and views about the use of action learning and its development. It includes listings of action learning-related events, book reviews and reports of conferences, and also promotes discussion through articles and correspondence.

- ***Meetings, conferences and workshops*:** Workshops and conferences are held regularly in the UK and the design of these is always participative, following a key principle of action learning, that people learn best with and from other people who are also learning.
- ***Network*:** With members in the UK and internationally, IFAL creates a network of people who wish to develop their own and others' knowledge and practice of action learning.

Further information from: www.ifal.org.uk or contact IFAL Administration Office:

18A Madeira Road
CLEVEDON
North Somerset
BS21 7TJ
UK

Global Forum on Leadership, Learning and Strategic Change

The Global Forum is a not-for-profit community of practice involving participants from major companies and organisations from around the world, who, in a collegial spirit, discuss strategic change, executive learning and organisation development. Originally titled the annual Global Forum on Executive Development and Business Driven Action Learning, it commenced in 1996. Attendance at the annual Global Forum is by invitation only and is restricted to no more than 100 participants. Sessions take place over a period of three and a half days and are informal and interactive. They have taken place in the USA, France, Australia, South Africa, Netherlands, Germany, China, Canada, Ireland, South Korea, Singapore, Japan, Switzerland, Sweden, Poland and the UK. One of the objectives is to continually develop and improve methods and techniques in the business-driven action learning field, although the events are not confined to that purpose.

More information is available at: www.globalforum-actionlearning.com Or from Yury Boshyk at yury@gel-net.com

World Institute for Action Learning (WIAL)

The WIAL is a not-for-profit international organisation dedicated to the advancement of a particular *'brand'* of action learning, associated with the work and writings of Professor Michael Marquardt, and within business and all community sectors. It has worked, often through affiliates, in many multinational private sector organisations, but also in some parts of the public sector. Very much a business-driven and *'bottom-line'* approach, the action learning set facilitator takes on the role of coach. It claims to be the *'only certifying body for action learning'*, which is somewhat less than accurate. WIAL can be contacted at:

World Institute for Action Learning
PO Box 7601 #83791
WASHINGTON DC 20044
USA
or at info@wial.org

International Management Centres and Revans University

The International Management Centres (IMC) or International Management Centres Association (IMCA) was created in 1964 at Buckingham in the UK and with the aim of being the leading global professional development body for career and continuing professional development through action learning. It set out to offer action learning qualification programmes delivered by global and local faculty and supported locally through face-to-face meetings. However, the UK's Education Reform Act of 1988 made the IMC/IMCA's programmes illegal and so in 1999 Revans University, sometimes known as the University of Action Learning (UAL) was formed, sponsored by IMC/IMCA and based in Vanuatu. It is the unaccredited degree-awarding body of IMC/IMCA. It has no physical campus and all its activities take place online.

Neither Revans University nor IMC/IMCA are recognised as a UK degree-awarding body or course provider and British universities do not accept qualifications accredited by Revans University. Since 2005 Revans University and IMC/IMCA have not been accredited by the United States Distance Education and Training Council (DETC).

For further information, contact:

IMC Buckingham Office
Marriotts
Castle Street
BUCKINGHAM
MK18 1BP
UK

Action Learning, Action Research Association, Inc (ALARA)

Originating in Australia, ALARA describes itself as a global network of programmes, institutions, professionals and people interested in using action learning and action research to generate collaborative learning, training, research and action to advance social change and to transform workplaces, schools, colleges, universities, communities, voluntary organisations, governments and businesses.

Its vision is that action learning and action research will be widely used and publicly shared by individuals and groups creating local and global change for the achievement of a more equitable, just, joyful, productive, peaceful and sustainable society. It aims to facilitate networking amongst members and others in projects, research, teaching or learning about action learning, action research and process management and related approaches.

Further information is available at: www.alarassociation.org

REFERENCE

1. H. Pocock, SQIFED: A new reflective model for action learning, *Journal of Paramedic Practice* 5 (3); 2013: 146–151.

FURTHER READING – HEALTH CARE

L. Abbott, Action learning as a tool to prepare supervisors of midwives, *British Journal of Midwifery* 19 (3); 2011: 185–189.

K. Aspinwall, *Evaluation Study: 18 Month Follow-Up of Phase 2 of The Department of Health Pathology Action Learning Programme* (Hathersage: ALSI Ltd, 2009).

C. Atkinson and A. Landrock, Using action learning sets to facilitate CPD in Uganda, *Occupational Therapy News* 2011: 38–40.

M. Attwood, Challenging from the margins into the mainstream: Improving renal services in a collaborative and entrepreneurial spirit, *Action Learning: Research & Practice* 4 (2); 2007: 191–198.

T. Balslev, Action learning in the paediatric neurology clinic, *Medical Education* 38 (5); 2004: 564–565.

A. Bamford-Wade and C. Moss, Transformational leadership and shared governance: An action study, *Journal of Nursing Management* 18 (7); 2010: 815–821.

A. Baquer and J. Craig, Action learning: Staff training based on evaluation of the services by the providers, *Journal of European Industrial Training* 2 (1); 1973: 43–55.

M. Barclay, *Better Together: Sharing Learning to Improve Care* (Petersfield: NHS Kidney Care, 2012).

E. Barnett and S. Ndeki, Action-based learning to improve district management: A case study from Tanzania, *International Journal of Health Planning & Management* 7 (4); 1992: 299–308.

D. Bazos, K. Schifferdecker, R. Fedrizzi, J. Hoebeke, L. Ruggles and Y. Goldsberry, Action learning collaboratives as a platform for community-based participatory research to advance obesity prevention, *Journal of Health Care for the Poor & Underserved* 24 (2); 2013: 61–79.

A. Beattie, Action learning for health on campus, in *Health-Promoting Universities*, eds. A. Tsouros, G. Dowding, J. Thompson and M. Dooris (Copenhagen: World Health Organisation (Europe), 1998), 45–55.

M. Bell, E. Coen, A. Coyne-Nevin, R. Egenton, A. Ellis and L. Moran, Experiences of an action learning set, *Practice Development in Health Care* 6 (4); 2007: 232–241.

L. Beniston, P. Ellwood, J. Gold J. Roberts and R. Thorpe, Innovation development: An action learning programme for medical scientists and engineers, *Action Learning: Research & Practice* 11 (3); 2014: 311–329.

L. Benson, *Evaluation of The SDO Networks and North West Strategic Health Authority Action Learning: September*, 2008 *To June, 2009*, NHS North West, 2009.

M. Bering, A personal journey into leadership, *Nursing Standard* 13 (4); 2006: 20–25.

J. Biggam, *Evaluating Online Action Learning Sets in The Development of Practitioner Skills* (Glasgow: Glasgow Caledonian University for NHS Education for Scotland, 2010).

F. Biley, W. Hilton, J. Phillips and M. Board, A brief report on an action learning group exploration of how older people adapt to change in later life, *Nursing Reports* 2 (1); 2012: 13–17.

B. Billington, B. Dickinson, B. Durkin, E. Grattage, M. Jones, B. McCallum, L Millward et al. *Action Learning in Hospitals for the Mentally Handicapped: Report by the Staff of the Whittington Hall Unit in Conjunction with Action Learning Projects International Ltd* (Southport: Action Learning Projects International Ltd, 1977).

F. Blackler and A. Kennedy, The design and evaluation of a leadership programme for experienced chief executives from the health sector, in *Action Learning, Leadership and Organisational Development in Public Services*, eds. C. Rigg and S. Richards (London: Routledge, 2006), pp. 79–99.

C. Blanchard and B. Carpenter, Experiences of action learning groups for public health sector managers in rural KwaZulu-Natal, South Africa, *Remote & Rural Health* 12 (2026); 2012: 1–11.

G. Boak, Enabling team learning in healthcare, *Action Learning: Research & Practice* 13 (2); 2016: 101–117.

M. Board and M. Symons, Community matron role development through action learning, *Primary Health Care* 17 (8); 2007: 19–22.

A. Booth, A. Sutton and L. Falzon, Working together: Supporting projects through action learning, *Health Information & Libraries Journal* 20 (4); 2003: 225–231.

D. Boston and M. Carter, Action learning for clinical governance *Organisations & People* 9 (1); 2002: 22–27.

D. Botham, D. Vick, S. Young and D. Clarke, *The Selection of Action Learning Set Facilitators for Primary Care Trusts Health Management* (London: NHS Modernisation Agency, 2003).

J. Bowerman, Leadership development through action learning: An executive monograph, *Leadership in Health Services* 16 (4); 2003: 6–14.

A. Breen, A. Langworthy, J. Worswick, P. Wilcock, D. Hettinga, D. Campion-Smith and E. Carr, *Using Collaborative Action Learning to Improve the Management of Back Pain in the Community* (Bournemouth: Bournemouth University/The Health Foundation, 2011.)

V. Breen, Action learning sets to support specialist screening practitioners, *Gut* 62 (Supplement); 2013: 261–262.

N. Bristow, Clinical leadership in the NHS: Evaluating change through action learning, in *Management Development: Perspectives from Research and Practice*, eds. R. Hill and J. Stewart (London: Routledge, 2007).

C. Brook, The role of the NHS in the development of Revans' action learning: Correspondence and contradiction in action learning development and practice, *Action Learning: Research & Practice* 7 (2); 2010: 181–192.

C. Brook, Action learning in health care, in *Action Learning and its Applications*, eds. R. Dilworth and Y. Boshyk (Basingstoke: Palgrave Macmillan, 2010).

N. Brooks and A. Moriarty, Development of a practice learning team in the clinical setting, *Nursing Standard* 20 (33); 2006: 41–44.

M. Brownlee and R. Foy, Evidence-based midwifery care: Evaluation of a pilot action learning programme, *Practice Midwife* 3 (1); 2000: 23–26.

F. Cantle, Tackling perinatal mental health among black and minority ethnic mothers, *Ethnicity & Inequalities in Health & Social Care* 3 (2); 2010: 38–43.

C. Carlson and J. Wright, *Enabling the Development of Public Health Networks: National Public Health Network Action Learning Set Programme: Summary Report* (Oxford: Public Health Resource Unit, Department of Health, 2004).

A. Chapman and R. Hosking, *Bridging the Gap: An Action Learning Approach to Improving Care Practice* (Stirling: Dementia Services Development Centre, University of Stirling, 2009).

S. Charman, M. McArthur, J. Davies and C. Burke, *'Access for All' Action Learning Sets: Evaluation Report* (CAMHS Consultants/Foundation For People With Learning Disabilities, 2007).

M. Chivers, Ordinary magic: Developing services for children with severe communication difficulties by engaging multiple voices, *Action Learning: Research & Practice* 2 (1); 2005: 7–26.

M. Chivers and A. Yates, Towards an ecology of organisation: The impact of an action learning strategy in an NHS trust, *Paper Presented at 1st International Conference On, Action Learning: Practices, Problems & Prospects*, Henley Management College, April, 2008.

Y. Cho, H. Bong and K. Jang, Action learning for developing nurses in South Korea, *International Journal of Human Resources Development & Management* 12 (4); 2012: 274–291.

A. Christiansen, C. Prescott and J. Ball, Learning in action: Developing safety improvement capabilities through action learning, *Nurse Education Today* 34 (2); 2014: 243–247.

A. Christiansen, L. Robson and C. Griffiths-Evans, Creating an improvement culture for enhanced patient safety: Service improvement learning in pre- registration education, *Journal of Nursing Management* 18 (7); 2010: 782–788.

K.-H. Chung and S.-G. Park, The effect of action learning-based teaching and learning strategies on the competency development of nursing students, *Advanced Science & Technology Letters (Healthcare & Nursing)* 104; 2015: 115–118.

K.-H. Chung and S.-G. Park, The effect of action learning-based teaching and learning strategies on metacognitive, problem-solving, interpersonal relations and team efficacy of nursing students, *International Journal of Service, Science & Technology* 8 (11); 2015: 65–74.

E. Clark, Action learning with young carers, *Action Learning: Research & Practice* 1 (1); 2004: 109–116.

E. Clark, L. Smith and G. Harvey, *Final Report of Evaluation of Action Learning for Improvement in the NHS* (Coventry: NHS Institute for Innovation & Improvement, 2009).

D. Clarke, *Evaluation of Practice: Action Learning Sets for Facilitators: Evaluative Report on the National Primary & Care Trust Transformational Change Action Learning Programme* (Revans Centre for Action Learning & Research, University of Salford for NHS Modernisation Agency, 2004).

D. Clarke and B. Allyson, *Action Learning for Continuing Professional Development* (Revans Centre for Action Learning & Research, University of Salford for Institute of Healthcare Management, 2003).

D. Clarke, E. Clarke, S. Young, D. Vick and D. Botham, The Selection of Action Learning Set Facilitators for Primary Care Trust Health Management (*Revans Centre for Action Learning & Research*, University of Salford for NHS Modernisation Agency, 2003).

N. Coghill and J. Stewart, The NHS: Myth, Monster or Service: Action Learning in Hospital (*Revans Centre for Action Learning & Research*, University of Salford, 1998).

A. Collin and J. Sturt, *Report of an Evaluation Study of an Action Learning Project in Hospitals for the Mentally Handicapped, North Derbyshire Health District* (Sheffield: Trent Regional Health Authority Organisation Development Unit, 1978).

D. Cortazzi and A. Baquer, *Action Learning: A Guide to its Use for Hospital Staff Based on a Pilot Study in Coordination in Hospitals for the Mentally Handicapped* (London: King Edwards Hospital Fund for London Hospital Centre, 1972).

L. Crofts, Learning from experience: Constructing critical case reviews for a leadership programme, *Intensive & Critical Care Nursing* 22 (5); 2006: 294–300.

G. Currie, The NHS: Myth, monster or service?: Action learning in hospital, *Management Learning* 30 (4); 1999: 507–508.

K. Currie, J. Biggam, J. Palmer and T. Corcoran, Participants' engagement with and reaction to the use of action learning sets to support advanced nursing role development, *Nurse Education Today* 32 (3); 2012: 267–272.

L. Curry and J. Farhall, The shift from psychiatric nurse to manager: The design, implementation and evaluation of an action learning programme, *International Journal for Therapeutic & Supportive Organisations* 16 (4); 1995: 215–228.

L. Dack, Action learning: A case study supporting clinical leadership development, in *Clinical Leadership: A Book of Readings*, ed. John Edmonstone (Chichester: Kingsham Press, 2005), pp. 151–162.

N. Davies, Grab a piece of the action, *Nursing Standard* 25 (48); 2011: 62–63.

C. Davis and J. Curzio, Avoiding the pitfalls of action learning, *Nurse Education in Practice* 3 (4); 2004: 183–184.

K. Davis, S. Brownie, F. Doran, S. Evans, M. Hutchinson, B. Mozolic-Staunton, S. Provost and R. Van Aken, Action learning enhances professional development of research supervisors: An Australian health science exemplar, *Nursing & Health Sciences* 14 (1); 2012: 102–108.

Department of Health. *Acting for Change: Transforming Pathology Services Through Action Learning* (London: Department of Health, 2008).

Department of Health. *Modernising from Within: Action Learning Solutions for Pathology: Learning from Phase 1 of the Pathology Action Learning Programme, 2005–2006* (London: Department of Health, 2007).

Department of Health. *Action Learning: Transforming Renal and Pathology Services* (London: Department of Health, 2006).

J. Dewing and J. Wright, A practice development project for nurses working with older people, *Practice Development in Healthcare* 2 (1); 2003: 13–28.

D. Dinkin and S. Frederick, Action learning projects used in public health leadership institutes, *Leadership in Health Services* 26 (1); 2013: 7–19.

O. Donnenburg, Network learning in an Austrian hospital – revisited, in *Action Learning in Practice*, Fourth edition, ed. M. Pedler (Aldershot: Gower Publishing, 2011).

K. Douglas, Taking action to close the nursing-finance gap: Learning from success, *Nursing Economics* 28 (4); 2010: 270–272.

J. Down and S. Hardy, Action learning: Positive impact on patient-centred, evidence-based care and cultural change? *Paper Presented at 6th International Conference on Practice Development, Action Research & Reflective Practice*, Edinburgh, 2006.

L. Doyle, Action learning: developing leaders and supporting change in a healthcare context, *Action Learning: Research & Practice* 11 (1); 2014: 64–71.

E. Dunne and F. Kelliher, Learning in action: Creating a community of inquiry in a healthcare organisation, *Action Learning: Research & Practice* 10 (2); 2013: 148–157.

G. Dunne R. Jooste and C. McCabe, The use of action learning as a strategy for improving pain management in the emergency department, *International Emergency Nursing* 22 (6); 2014: 172–176.

L. Dunphy, G. Proctor, R. Bartlett, M. Haslam and C. Wood, Reflections and learning from using action learning sets in a healthcare education setting, *Action Learning: Research & Practice* 7 (3); 2010: 303–314.

S. Du Toit, A. Wilkinson and K. Adam, Role of research in occupational therapy clinical practice: Applying action learning and action research in pursuit of evidence-based practice, *Australian Occupational Therapy Journal* 57 (5); 2010: 318–330.

J. Edmonstone, The relevance of action learning to problem-solving and manager development in the NHS, *Health Services Manpower Review* 8 (1); 1982: 16–19.

J. Edmonstone, Action learning as a developmental practice for clinical leadership, *International Journal of Clinical Leadership* 16 (2); 2008: 59–64.

J. Edmonstone, When action learning doesn't 'Take': reflections on the DALEK Programme, *Action Learning: Research & Practice* 7 (1); 2010: 89–97.

J. Edmonstone, *Action Learning in Healthcare: A Practical Handbook* (Milton Keynes: Radcliffe Publishing, 2011).

J. Edmonstone and H. Mackenzie, Practice Development and Action Learning, *Practice Development in Health Care* 4 (1); 2005: 24–32.

J. Edmonstone and J. Robson, Blending-in: The contribution of action learning to a masters programme in human resources in health, *International Journal of Human Resource Development & Management* 13 (1); 2013: 61–75.

J. Edmonstone and J. Robson, Action learning on the edge: Contributing to a masters programme in human resources for health, *Action Learning: Research & Practice* 11 (3); 2014: 361–374.

T. Emerson, V. Morley and C. Bell, ALS support for GP projects, *Organisations & People* 6 (3); 1999: 17–23.

Faculty of Public Health Medicine, *Learning Sets: A Tool for Developing a Multi-Agency, Multi-Professional Approach to Public Health* (London: Public Health & Primary Care Group, 2001).

P. Finlay and C. Marples, Experience in using action learning sets to enhance information management and technology strategic thinking in the UK National Health Service, *Journal of Management Studies* 7 (2); 1998: 165–184.

N. Foss and A. Bardsen, Playful reflection: an investigation into the kindergarten project 'Play in Physiotherapy with Children', *Action Learning: Research & Practice* 10 (2); 2013: 107–123.

R. Foy, N. Tidy and S. Hollis, Inter-professional learning in primary care: Lessons from an action learning programme, *British Journal of Clinical Governance* 7 (1); 2002: 40–44.

P. French, P. Callaghan, S. Dudley-Brown, E. Holroyd and K. Sellick, The effectiveness of tutorials in behavioural sciences for nurses: An action learning project, *Nurse Education Today* 18 (2); 1998: 116–124.

D. Freshwater, Managing practice innovations in prison health services, *Nursing Times* 102 (7); 2006: 32.

V. Gibbs and J. Hobbs, Implementing a new style of learning in a taught post- graduate medical ultrasound programme: Reflections on the first year, *Ultrasound* 17 (2); 2009: 85–89.

G. Giles, Report on accreditation learning sets in the West Midlands Region of the NHS, *Health Libraries Review* 17 (4); 2000: 181–188.

I. Graham, Reflective practice: Using the action learning group mechanism, *Nurse Education Today* 15 (1); 1995: 28–32.

I. Graham and C. Partlow, Introducing and developing nurse leadership through a learning set approach, *Nurse Education Today* 24 (6); 2004: 459–465.

W. Griffiths, Action learning for quality assurance – a diary: Part 1, *International Journal of Health Care Quality Assurance* 1 (3); 1988: 29–31.

W. Griffiths and R. Gourlay, Action learning for quality assurance—a diary: Part 2, *International Journal of Health Care Quality Assurance* 2 (1); Research Paper, 1989.

J. Habey, Improving patient outcomes through action learning, *Paper Presented at 6th International Conference on Practice Development, Action Research & Reflective Practice*, Edinburgh, 2006.

M. Haith and K. Whittingham, How to use action learning sets to support nurses, *Nursing Times* 108 (18/19); 2012: 12–14.

J. Hardacre and J. Keep, From intent to impact: Developing clinical leaders for service improvement, *Learning in Health & Social Care* 2 (3); 2003: 169–176.

S. Harpur, Leadership collaboration during health reform: An action learning approach with an interagency group of Executives in Tasmania, *Australian Health Review* 36 (2); 2012: 136–139.

R. Harrison and S. Miller, The contribution of clinical directors to the strategic capability of the organisation, *British Journal of Management* 10 (1); 1999: 23.

R. Harrison, S. Miller and A. Gibson, Doctors in management – Part 2: Getting into action, *Executive Development* 6 (4); 1993a: 3–7.

R. Harrison, S. Miller and A. Gibson, Doctors in management – Part 1: Two into one won't go – or will it? *Executive Development* 6 (2); 1993b: 9–13.

F. Heidari, Evaluation of action learning groups within pre-registration nurse education, *Paper Presented at First Annual UK & USA Conference on the Scholarship of Teaching & Learning*, London, 2001.

F. Heidari and K. Galvin, Action learning groups: Can they help students develop their knowledge and skills? *Nurse Education in Practice* 3 (1); 2002: 49–55.

A. Hewison, F. Badger and T. Swani, Leading end of life care: An action learning approach in nursing homes, *International Journal of Palliative Care* 17 (3); 2011: 135–141.

F. Hicks, K. Winterburn and A. Edwards, Action learning as a novel approach to change clinical practice, *BMJ Supportive & Palliative Care* 4 (1); 2014.

J. Hockley, J. Levy, R. Heal and J. Kinley, The use of action learning sets to enhance facilitation of the gold standards framework in care homes' end of life care programme: The intervention arm of a cluster randomised control trial, London, St Christopher's Hospice, *Paper Presented at 19th International Congress on Palliative Care*, Montreal, Canada, 2012.

A. Hughes, P. Elson and I. Govier, Developing practice nurses' leadership skills, *Practice Nursing* 17 (8); 2006: 376–378.

V. Jackson, Using action learning to improve the quality of care in hospitals, *American Journal of Medical Quality* 18 (3); 2003: 104–107.

V. Jackson, Medical quality management: The case for action learning as a quality initiative, *Leadership in Health Services* 17 (2); 2004: 1–8.

G. Jacobs, The development of critical being? Reflection and reflexivity in an action learning programme for health promotion practitioners in the Netherlands, *Action Learning: Research & Practice* 5 (3); 2008: 221–235.

G. Jacobs, 'Take control or lean back?': Barriers to practicing empowerment in health promotion, *Health Promotion Practitioner* 12 (1); 2011: 94–101.

K. Jang, Action learning in the hospital: A case of Chonnam National University Hospital, *HRD Monthly*, 2011: 56–59.

K-S. Jang, N-Y. Kim and H. Park, Effects of an action learning-based creative problem-solving course for nursing students, *Journal of Korean Academy of Nursing Administration* 20 (5); 2014: 47–53.

E. Jenkins, G. Mabbett, A. Surridge, J. Warring and E. Gwynne, A cooperative inquiry into action learning and praxis development in a module for community nurses, *Qualitative Health Research* 19 (9); 2009: 1303–1320.

L. Jenstad and M. Donnelly, Hearing care for elders: A personal reflection on participatory action learning with primary care providers, *American Journal of Audiology* 10; 2015: 23–30.

A. Jones and T. Prescott, Action learning: A new way of problem solving in perioperative settings, in *Core Topics in Operating Department Practice: Leadership and Management*, eds. B. Smith, P. Rawling, P. Wicker and C. Jones (Cambridge: Cambridge University Press, 2009).

K. Jones, J. Bunker, S. Heywood, J. Van Tromp and W. Brown, Action learning to provide continuing professional development, *Nurse Prescribing*, 3 (4); 2005: 156–158.

J. Kellie, E. Henderson, B. Milsom and H. Crawley, Leading change in tissue viability best practice: An action learning programme for link nurse practitioners, *Action Learning: Research & Practice* 7 (2); 2010: 213–219.

J. Kellie, B. Milsom and E. Henderson, Leadership through action learning: A bottom-up approach to 'best practice', in 'Infection Prevention and Control', In A UK NHS Trust, *Public Money & Management* (July); 2012: 289–296.

J. Kells, Action learning in the health and social services in Northern Ireland, *Hospital & Health Services Review* 81 (2); 1985: 69–71.

M. Kelly and N. Hooke, Help for the helpless: The journey through action learning to becoming practice developers, *Paper Presented at 6th International Conference on Practice Development*, Action Research & Reflective Practice, Edinburgh, 2006.

Y-M. Kim and Y-H. Kim, Development and evaluation of action learning in clinical practice of nursing management, *Journal of Korea Contents Association* 10 (6); 2010: 312–322.

C. Kirrane, Using action learning in reflective practice, *Professional Nurse* 16 (5); 2001: 102–105.

S. Lamont, S. Brunero and R. Russell, An exploratory evaluation of an action learning set within a mental health service, *Nurse Education in Practice* 10 (5); 2010: 298–302.

S. Laverty, Helping doctors to solve problems, *BMJ Career Focus* 329; 2004: 59–60.

A. Learmonth, Action learning as a tool for developing networks and building evidence-based practice in public health, *Action Learning: Research & Practice* 2 (1); 2005: 97–104.

A. Learmonth and M. Pedler, Auto action learning: A tool for policy change? Building capacity across the developing regional system to improve health in the North East of England, *Health Policy* 68 (2); 2004: 169–181.

K. Lee and C. Porteous, Case loading: Students solve their own problems using action learning, *British Journal of Midwifery* 18 (9); 2010: 603–609.

N. Lee, Action learning: A beginner's guide to the principles of action learning, *Nursing Times Learning Curve* 3 (6); 1999a: 2–3.

N. Lee, Thinking reflectively: Solutions through action learning, *Nursing Times* 49; 1999b: 54–55.

S. Leggat, C. Balding and J. Anderson, Empowering health care managers in Australia: An action learning approach, *Health Services Management Research* 24 (4); 2011: 196–202.

S. Leggat, C. Balding and D. Schiftan, Developing clinical leaders: The impact of an action learning mentoring programme for advanced practice nurses, *Journal of Clinical Nursing* 24 (11–12); 2015: 1576–1584.

U. Lehmann and L. Gilson, Action learning for health system governance: The reward and challenge of co-production, *Health Policy & Planning* 30 (8); 2015: 957–963.

R. Lewis, Modernising pathology: What can action learning do for you? *Royal College of Pathologists Bulletin* 133; 2006: 14–16.

M. Lorentzon, The NHS: Myth, monster or service? Action learning in hospital, *Journal of Nursing Management* 6 (5); 1998: 321.

L. Lynch and E. Verner, Building a clinical leadership community to drive improvement: A multi-case educational study to inform twenty-first century clinical commissioning, Professional capability and patient care, *Education for Primary Care* 24 (1); 2013: 22–28.

M. Lynch and N. McFetridge, Practice leaders programme: Entrusting and enabling general practitioners to lead change to improve patient experience, *The Permanente Journal* 15 (1); 2011: 17–43.

A. Machin and P. Pearson, Action learning sets in a nursing and midwifery practice learning context: A realistic evaluation, *Nurse Education in Practice* 14 (4); 2014: 410–416.

R. Mann, K. Ball and G. Watson, Mentoring for NHS general practitioners: A prospective pilot study of an action learning approach, *Education in Primary Care* 22 (4); 2011: 235–240.

A. Marlow, C. Spratt and A. Reilly, Collaborative action learning: A professional development model for educational innovation in nursing, *Nurse Education in Practice* 8; 2008: 184–189.

F. McAlinden, Using action research and action learning (ARAL) to develop a response to the abuse of older people in a healthcare context, *Journal of Work- Applied Management* 7 (1); 2015: 38–51.

M. McAndrew, Use of an action learning model to create a dental faculty development programme, *Journal of Dental Education* 74 (5); 2010: 517–523.

D. McAree and E. Scott, Action learning as an improved method for continuing professional development for pharmacists providing women's health care advice, *International Journal of Pharmacy Practice* 9; 2001: 82.

B. McCormack, C. O'Connell and C. Kerr, *A Framework for Evaluating Action Learning in the Royal Hospitals Trust* (Belfast: Royal Hospitals Trust, 2003).

C. McKenzie, Enhancing the care of the older person through action learning, *Paper Presented at 6th International Conference on Practice Development, Action Research & Reflective Practice*, Edinburgh, 2006.

M. McNamara, G. Fealy, M. Casey, T. O'Connor, D. Patton, L. Doyle and C. Quinlan, Mentoring, coaching and action learning: Interventions in a national clinical leadership programme, *Journal of Clinical Nursing* 23 (17/18); 2014: 2533–2541.

M. Mead, C. Yearley, C. Lawrence and C. Rogers, Action learning: A learning and teaching method in the preparation programme for supervisors of midwives, *Action Learning: Research & Practice* 3 (2); 2006: 175–186.

J. Moore, W. Neithercut, A. Mellors, D. Manning, C. Makin, H. Jones, R. Alman and M. Al-Bachari, Making the new deal for junior doctors happen, *British Medical Journal* 308; 1994: 1553–1555.

S. Nash and J. Scammell, How to use coaching and action learning to support mentors in the workplace, *Nursing Times* 106; 2010: 20–23.

R. Newton and M. Wilkinson, When the talking is over: Using action learning, *Health Manpower Management* 21 (5); 1995: 34–39.

D. Nicolini, M. Sher, S. Childerstone and M. Gorli, In search of the 'Structure that Reflects': Promoting organisational reflection in a UK health authority, *Paper Presented at the 5th International Conference on Organisational Learning & Knowledge*, University of Lancaster, 2003.

D. Nicolini, M. Sher, S. Childerstone and M. Gorli, In search of the 'Structure that Reflects': Promoting organisational reflection practices in a UK Health Authority, in *Organising Reflection*, eds. Mike Reynolds and Russ Vince (Aldershot: Ashgate, 2004).

Office for Health Management, Action learning guide, Dublin, Irish Republic, 2003.
Onyett, S. Leadership for change, *Mental Health Review* 7 (4); 2002: 20–23.

M. Pedler, On the right course, *Health Management* 10 (2); 2006: 24–25.

M. Pedler and C. Abbott, Am I doing it right? facilitating action learning for service improvement, *Leadership in Health Services* 21 (3); 2008a: 185–199.

M. Pedler and C. Abbott, Lean and learning: Action learning for service improvement, *Leadership in Health Services* 21 (2); 2008b: 87–98.

M. Pedler and J. Boutall, *Action Learning for Change: A Resource Book for Managers and Other Professionals* (Bristol: National Health Service Training Directorate, 1992).

M. Pedler, R. Lewis, S. Mousdale, C. Jones, N. Pritchard, D. Milford, D. Fisher and S. Marks, Renal action learning sets: A report of progress so far, *British Journal of Renal Medicine* 13 (3); 2008: 27–31.

D. Phelan and G. Birchall, Action learning groups and cultural change in hospitals, *Health Care & Informatics Review* 5 (4); 2001.

M. Plack, M. Driscoll, M. Marquez and L. Greenberg, Peer-facilitated virtual action learning: Critical incidents during a paediatric clerkship, *Academic Paediatrics* 10 (2); 2010: 146–152.

M. Plack, H. Dunfee, A. Rindflesch and M. Driscoll, Virtual action learning sets: A model for facilitating reflection in the clinical setting, *Journal of Physical Therapy Education* 22 (2); 2008: 60–67.

H. Pocock, SQIFED: A new reflective model for action learning, *Journal of Paramedic Practice* 5 (3); 2013: 146–151.

D. Rayner, H. Chisholm and H. Appleby, Developing leadership through action learning, *Nursing Standard* 16 (29); 2002: 37–39.

R. Revans (Ed.), *Hospitals: Communication, Choice and Change: The Hospital Internal Communications Project Seen from Within* (London: Tavistock Publications, 1972).

R. Revans, Helping each other to help the helpless: An essay in self-organisation: Part 1, *Kybernetes* 4; 1975a: 149–155.

R. Revans, Helping each other to help the helpless: An essay in self-organisation: Part 2, *Kybernetes* 4; 1975b: 205–211.

R. Revans, *Action Learning in Hospitals: Diagnosis and Therapy* (Maidenhead: McGraw-Hill, 1976).

R. Revans, Action learning takes a health cure, *Education & Training* 20 (11); 1978: 295–299.

R. Revans, Action learning; The cure is started (at west Middlesex hospital, Britain), *Management Decision* 21 (4); 1983: 11–16.

J. Richardson, R. Ainsworth, R. Allison, J. Billyard, R. Corley and J. Viner, Using an action learning set to support the nurse and allied health professional consultant role, *Action Learning: Research & Practice* 5 (1); 2008: 65–78.

K. Rivas and S. Murray, Our shared experience of implementing action learning sets in an acute clinical nursing setting: Approach taken and lessons learned, *Contemporary Nurse* 35 (2); 2010: 182–187.

C. Roberts and D. Coghlan, Concentric collaboration: A model of leadership development for healthcare organisations, *Action Learning: Research & Practice* 8 (3); 2011: 231–252.

K. Rogan, The introduction of action learning into a midwifery curriculum, *Paper Presented at Bournemouth University Collaborative Conference*, Bournemouth, 2003.

Z. Rojas, P. Sandiford, E. Coyle and P. Allen, Action learning: Is this the way to train health managers in developing countries? *Education in Medical Health* 29 (2); 1995: 189–205.

D. Rosenbaum, E. More and P. Steane, Action learning intervention as a change management strategy in the disablement services sector: A case study, *ALAR Journal* 18 (2); 2012.

J. Rudman, J. Bennis and C. Jones, Using action learning in practice development, *Paper Presented at 6th International Conference on Practice Development*, Action Research & Reflective Practice, Edinburgh, 2006.

K. Schachter, M. Ingram, L. Jacobs, J. De Zapien, H. Hafter and S. Carvajal, Developing an action learning community advocacy/leadership training program for community health workers and their agencies to reduce health disparities in Arizona border communities, *Journal of Health Disparities Research & Practice*, 7 (2); 2014: 34–49.

A. Scowcroft, The problem with dissecting a frog (Is that when you are finished it doesn't really look like a frog anymore), in *Clinical Leadership: A Book of Readings*, eds. J. Edmonstone (Chichester: Kingsham Press, 2005), pp. 271–291.

C. Sikorski, M. Lakhanpaul, A. Costello and M. Heys, A systemic review: 'Can participatory action learning methods improve health outcomes in high-income countries?', *Archives of Disease in Childhood* 99 (1); 2014: 197–198.

A. Smith and J. Greaves, Evaluation of a series of action learning sets designed to provide professional development opportunities for nurses in general practice, *Paper Presented at Royal College of Nursing International Nursing Research Conference*, York, 2006.

M. Spurrell, Consultant learning groups in psychiatry: Report on a pilot study, *Psychiatric Bulletin* 24; 2000: 390–392, Royal College of Psychiatrists.

M. Striano, A. Romano and M. Strollo, Reframing professional challenges through action learning conversations in medical organisations, *Proceedings of XII International Transformative Learning Conference 'Engaging at The Intersections'*, Tacoma, Washington, 2016.

D. Sutton, *Action Learning in Hospitals for the Mentally Handicapped* (Southport: ALP International Ltd, 1977a).

D. Sutton, Improving services for the mentally handicapped, *Action Learning Trust Newsletter* 1; 1977b.

T. Swani, The impact of the action learning approach in nursing homes, *BMJ Supportive & Palliative Care* 1; 2011: 208–209.

J. Thomas and G. Etheridge, Using action learning to support and develop the role of matrons, *Nursing Times* 100 (34); 2004: 36–38.

D. Towell and K. Barnard, *Towards an Action Learning Programme for the Development of Senior NHS Managers* (Leeds: Nuffield Centre for Health Service Studies, University of Leeds, 1976).

J. Traeger and C. Norgate, A safe place to stay sharp: Action learning meets cooperative inquiry in service of NHS OD capacity building, *Action Learning: Research & Practice* 12 (2); 2015: 197–207.

S. Walia and D. Marks-Maran, Leadership development through action learning sets: An evaluation study, *Nurse Education in Practice* 14 (6); 2014: 612–619.

M. Walker, B. Bromley and M. Mazaka, The use of action learning sets to enhance students' learning experiences during their dissertation project", *Paper Presented at Royal College of Nursing Education Forum Conference*, Harrogate, 2012.

E. Walsh and A. Bee, Developing a learning environment in prison health care, *International Journal of Practice Development* 2 (1); 2012: 1–15.

E. Walsh and D. Freshwater, Managing practice innovations in prison health care services, *Nursing Times* 102 (7); 2006: 32.

S. Walsh and C. Fegan, Action learning: Facilitating real change for part-time occupational therapy students, *Action Learning: Research & Practice* 4 (2); 2007: 137–152.

A. Waugh, L. McNay, B. Dewar and M. McCaig, Supporting the development of interpersonal skills in nursing, in an undergraduate mental health curriculum: Reaching the parts other strategies do not reach, *Nurse Education Today* 34 (9); 2014: 1232–1237.

C. Wedderburn, T. Battcock, M. Masding and S. Scallan, A pilot learning set for newly appointed GPS and hospital consultants, *Education for Primary Care* 23 (1); 2012: 47–49.

G. Weiland, *Improving Health Care Management: Organisation Development and Organisation Change*. (Ann Arbor, Michigan: Health Administration Press, 1981).

G. Weiland and H. Leigh (Eds.), *Changing Hospitals: A Report on The Hospital Internal Communications Project* (London: Tavistock Publications, 1971).

S. Willis, Student paramedics' perceptions of action learning: A mixed-methods study, *Journal of Paramedic Practice* 6 (12); 2014: 626–632.

D. Wilson and H. Jones, Working with GPS and hospital consultants on developing clinical leadership in a health community, in *Clinical Leadership: A Book of Readings*, eds. J. Edmonstone (Chichester: Kingsham Press, 2005), pp. 183–192.

V. Wilson, A. Ho and R. Walsh, Participatory action research and action learning: Changing clinical practice in nursing handover and communication, *Journal of Children's & Young People's Nursing* 2; 2007: 85–92.

V. Wilson, P. Keachie and M. Engelsmann, Putting the action into learning: The experience of an action learning set, *Collegian: Journal of The Royal College of Nursing Australia* 10 (3); 2003: 22–26.

V. Wilson, B. McCormack and G. Ives, Parallels of learning: The experience of an action learning set, *Educational Action Research* 14 (3); 2006: 35–42.

V. Wilson, B. McCormack and G. Ives, Developing healthcare practice through action learning: Individual and group journeys, *Action Learning: Research & Practice* 5 (1); 2008: 21–38.

V. Wilson, R. Walsh and A. Ho, Using action research and action learning to support and facilitate a change in nursing handover, *Journal of Children's and Young People's Nursing* 1 (1); 2007: 85–92.

T. Winkless, Yorkshire puts thoughts into action learning, *Health Service Manpower Review* 13 (3); 1987: 22–23.

K. Winterburn and F. Hicks, A mirror in which to practice: Using action learning to change end-of-life care, *Action Learning: Research & Practice* 9 (3); 2012: 307–315.

S. Young, E. Nixon, D. Hinge, J. McFadyen, V. Wright, P. Lambert, C. Pilkington and C. Newsome, Action learning: A tool for the development of strategic skills for nurse consultants, *Journal of Nursing Management* 18 (1); 2010: 105–110.

FURTHER READING: SOCIAL & COMMUNITY CARE (INCLUDING MULTI-AGENCY WORKING)

C. Abbott, L. Burtney and C. Wall, Building capacity in social care: An evaluation of a national programme of action learning facilitator development, *Action Learning: Research & Practice* 10 (2); 2013: 168–177.

C. Abbott and C. Mayes, Action learning for professionals: A new approach to practice, *Action Learning: Research & Practice* 11 (1); 2014: 72–80.

C. Abbott and P. Taylor, *Action Learning in Social Work* (London: Sage, 2013).

M. Baldwin and H. Burgess, Enquiry and action learning and practice placements, *Social Work Education* 11 (3); 1992: 36–44.

K. Ball, Action learning: Creating a space for multi-agency reflexivity to complement case management, *Practice* 25 (5); 2013: 335–347.

A. Baquer, *Project on Coordination of Services for the Mentally Handicapped* (London: King Edward's Hospital Fund for London, 1972).

A. Baquer and R. Revans, *But Surely that is Their Job? A Study in Practical Cooperation Through Action Learning* (Southport: ALP International Ltd, 1973).

S. Bell, M. Mattern and M. Telin, Community action learning, *Journal of Political Science Education* 3 (1); 2009: 61–78.

G. Bentley, F. McDonnell and H. Zutshi, *Action Learning for New Ways of Working Programme Evaluation* (London: Skills for Care, 2008).

S. Binns and I. McGill, Action learning at the London borough of eating, in *Reflective Learning in Practice*, eds. A. Brocklebank, I. McGill and N. Beech (Aldershot: Gower, 2002).

M. Bloodworth, Moving from opportunism to expediency when introducing action learning into an organisation, *Action Learning: Research & Practice* 11 (3); 2014: 352–360.

S. Bray, M. Preston-Shoot and T. Marrable, *Law Learning in Action: An Action Learning Project to Evaluate Processes and Outcomes of Using Law E-Learning Objects in Social Work Education* (Brighton: University of Bedfordshire/University of Sussex for Social Care Institute for Excellence, 2011).

K. Broughton, D. Jarvis and R. Farnell, Using action learning sets for more effective collaboration: The 'managing complex regeneration' programme, *Learning & Teaching in Higher Education* 4 (2); 2010: 16–21.

H. Burgess and S. Jackson, Enquiry and action learning: A new approach to social work education, *Social Work Education* 9 (3); 1990: 3–19.

H. Burgess and J. Reynolds, Preparing for social work with refugees using enquiry and action learning, *Social Work Education* 14 (4); 1996: 58–73.

R. Burgess, Reflective practice: Action learning sets for managers in social work, *Social Work Education* 18 (3); 1999: 257–270.

D. Burns, *Action Learning for Directors of Social Services* (Bristol, School of Policy Studies, Bristol University, 2001).

P. Candea, O. Lancaster, A. Morrow, K. Riddell and M. Watson, *Evaluation Report: Communities With a Common Cause Action Learning Programme* (Glasgow: Common Cause for Scotland, 2014).

L. Carson, Action learning teams: Building bridges within a local council, *Journal of Workplace Learning* 9 (5); 1997: 148–152.

J. Coates, An action learning approach to performance review and development: A case history from the London borough of Brimley, *Industrial & Commercial Training* 18 (4); 1986: 23–28.

D. Coghlan and P. Coughlan, Developing organisational learning capabilities through inter-organisational action learning, in *Current Topics in Management*, eds. M. Rahim, R. Golembiewski and K. MacKenzie, . (New Brunswick, NJ: Transaction, 2002), 7; pp. 24-27.

D. Coghlan and P. Coughlan, Action learning in inter-organisational sets, in *Action Learning, Leadership and Organisational Development in Public Services*, eds. C. Rigg and S. Richards (Abingdon: Routledge, 2006).

K. Corfield and M. Penney, Action learning in the community, in *Action Learning in Practice*, First edition, eds. Mike Pedler (Aldershot: Gower Publishing, 1983).

P. Coughlan and D. Coghlan, Action learning: Towards a framework in inter- organisational settings, *Action Learning: Research & Practice* 1 (1); 2004: 43–61.

H. Cramer, G. Dewulf and H. Voordijk, Lessons learned from applying action research to support strategy formation processes in long-term care networks, *Action Learning: Research & Practice* 12 (2); 2015: 166–194.

B. Cranwell, Action learning in the community, in *Action Learning in Practice*, First edition, eds. Mike Pedler (Aldershot: Gower Publishing, 1983).

G. Curtis-Jenkins and J. White, Action learning: A tool to improve inter-professional collaboration and promote change, *Journal of Inter-Professional Care* 8 (3); 1994: 265–273.

R. Dalrymple and P. Smith, Use of action learning with inter-professional cohorts on a leadership and management, *Learning & Teaching in Higher Education* 4 (2); 2010: 155–158.

H. David, Action learning for police officers in high crack areas, *Action Learning: Research & Practice* 3 (2); 2006: 189–196.

I. De Loo, An action learning failure in a Dutch municipality, *Public Administration Quarterly* 32 (2); 2008: 174–192.

S. Douglas and T. Machin, A model for setting up interdisciplinary collaborative working in groups: Lessons from an experience of action learning, *Journal of Psychiatric & Mental Health Nursing* 11; 2004: 189–193.

J. Edmonstone and H. Flanagan, A flexible friend: Action learning in the context of a multi-agency organisation development programme, *Action Learning: Research & Practice* 4 (2); 2007: 199–209.

J. Fardell, Bringing learning to life: A user-led action learning model, *Journal of Integrated Care* 11 (2); 2003: 36–42.

K. Faull, L. Hartley and T. Kalliath, Action learning: Developing a learning culture in a interdisciplinary rehabilitation team, *OD Journal* 23 (3); 2005: 39–52.

D. Foley, Developing citizen leaders through action learning, *Action Learning: Research & Practice* 3 (1); 2006: 79–87.

P. Fox, C. Rigg and M. Willis, Supporting organisational turnaround in local authorities, in *Action Learning, Leadership and Organisational Development in Public Services*, eds. Clare Rigg and Sue Richards (London: Routledge, 2006).

S. Gibbs, J. Gold and M. Cuthbert, Open space to the community: Action learning at a community level, *Action Learning: Research & Practice* 7 (1); 2010: 111–116.

J. Hunter, Leadership and engagement in South Cambridgeshire district council, *Action Learning: Research & Practice* 10 (1); 2013: 69–74.

C. Kagan, R. Lawthorn, A. Siddiquee, P. Duckett and K. Knowles, Community psychology through community action learning, in *Social Change in Solidarity: Community Perspectives and Approaches*, eds. A. Bokszczanin (Poland: Wydawnictwo University Press, 2007).

D. Kimoto, Transformational service and action learning: The sustainability of civic engagement, *Journal of Public Affairs Education* 17 (1); 2011: 27–43.

R. King, Enhancing the practice of social work, *Action Learning: Research & Practice* 13 (2); 2016: 168–175.

D. Langley and R. Watts, Women reaching women: Using action learning to help address seemingly intractable and large scale social issues, *Action Learning: Research & Practice* 7 (2); 2010: 207–211.

S. Leach and S. Hopgood, Cross-sector action learning for leaders, *International Journal of Leadership in Public Services* 2 (1); 2006: 38–42.

M. Lindeman, Using action learning for developing staff skills in interviewing children in child protection: a reflection on practice, *ALAR Journal* 13 (1); 2008: 53–64.

K. Lowe, Introducing action learning in local government: A new facilitator's experience, *Action Learning: Research & Practice* 7 (1); 2010: 83–87.

M. Lyons and R. Clare, Local authority chief executive action learning sets, in *Action Learning: Leadership and Organisation Development in Public Services*, eds. C. Rigg and S. Richards (Abingdon: Routledge, 2006).

P. Mann, K. Rummery and S. Pritchard, Supporting inter-organisational partnerships in the public sector: The role of joined-up action learning and research, *Public Management Review* 6 (3); 2004: 417–439.

S. Maslin-Prothero, S. Ashby and A. Rout, *Using an Action Learning Research Approach to Evaluate and Develop Inter-Professional Working Among Health and Social Care Staff, Particularly in Relation to the Care of Older People* (Keele: University of Keele, 2007).

F. McDonnell and H. Zutshi, *Learning to Transform Services: A Guide to Action Learning* (Skills for Care: London, 2009).

T. Morrison, *Staff Supervision in Social Care: An Action Learning Approach* (Harlow: Longman, 1993).

J. Muskett, From action learning to bonding social capital? The potential of action learning sets among isolated rural clergy, *Rural Theology* 14; 2016: 25–43.

J. Muskett and A. Village, Action learning sets and social capital: Ameliorating the burden of clergy isolation in one rural diocese, *Action Learning: Research & Practice* 13 (3); 2016.

NACVS, *Action Learning for Managers: Final Report, Plus Action Learning Matters* (Sheffield: National Association of Councils for Voluntary Service, 2004).

G. Overton, D. Kelly, P. McCalister, J. Jones and R. MacVicar, The practice- based small group learning approach: Making evidence-based practice come alive for learners, *Nurse Education Today* 29 (6); 2009: 671–675.

M. Pedler, C. Abbot, C. Brook and J. Burgoyne, *Improving Social Work Practice Through Critically Reflective Action Learning* (Leeds: Skills for Care, 2014).

J. Pettit, Getting to grips with power: Action learning for social change in the UK, *IDS Bulletin* 43 (3); 2012: 11–26.

J. Randall, P. Cowley and P. Tomlinson, Overcoming barriers to effective practice in child care, *Child & Family Social Work* 5 (4); 2000: 343.

B. Redmond, *Reflection in Action: Developing Reflective Practice in Health & Social Services.* (Aldershot: Ashgate, 2004).

R. Revans and A. Baquer, *I Thought They Were Supposed to be Doing That: A Comparative Study of Coordination of Services for the Mentally Handicapped in Seven Local Authorities* (London: The Hospital Centre, 1972).

J. Richardson and J. Grose, An action learning approach to partnership in community development: A reflection on the research process, *Action Learning: Research & Practice* 10 (3); 2013: 254–263.

C. Rigg, Action learning in the public service system: Issues, tensions and a future agenda, in *Action Learning: Leadership and Organisation Development in Public Services*, eds. C. Rigg and S. Richards (Abingdon: Routledge, 2006).

R. Sanders and L. McKeown, Promoting community through action learning in a 3D virtual world, *International Journal of Social Sciences* 2 (1); 2008: 50–55.

Scottish Government, *Guidance for Action Learning in Community Engagement: Based on The Experience of the Better Community Engagement Demonstration Project in Moray (2009–2011)* (Edinburgh: Scottish Government, 2012).

C. Sharpe, *Action Learning for Social Enterprises: Evaluation of Action Learning Group* (Edinburgh: Social Firms Scotland, 2005).

C. Skehill, Using a peer action learning approach in the implementation of communication and information technology in social work education, *Social Work Education: The International Journal* 22 (2); 2003: 177–190.

I. Taylor, Enquiry and action learning, in *Reflective Learning for Social Work*, eds. N. Gould and I. Taylor (Aldershot: Arena, 1996).

I. Taylor, Enquiry and action learning: Empowerment in social work, in *Educating Social Workers in a Changing Policy Context*, eds. M. Preston-Shoot and S. Jackson (London: Whiting & Birch, 1996).

P. West, Blackburn with Darwen action learning set: A model for improving the interface between inpatient and community teams, *Mental Health Review* 10 (1); 2005: 22–25.

P. Westoby, Reflections on community-based action learning with Vanuatu leaders: Building capacity for sustainable peace-building, in *From Theory to Practice: Context in Praxis (Proceedings from 5th Action Learning, Action Research & 12th Participatory Action Research 2010 World Congress)*, ed. S. Goff, (Melbourne: ALARA, 2013).

M. Willis, Partnership action learning, in *Action Learning, Leadership and Organisational Development in Public Services*, eds. C. Rigg and S. Richards (London: Routledge, 2006).

M. Willis, Tension, risk and conflict: Action learning journeys with four public sector partnership teams, *Action Learning: Research & Practice* 9 (2); 2012: 167–176.

V. Willis, Action learning, community and civil society, in *Action Learning and its Applications*, eds. R. Dilworth, and Y. Boshyk (Basingstoke: Palgrave Macmillan, 2010).

O. Zuber-Skerrit and R. Teare, *Action Learning for Community Development: Learning and Development for a Better World* (Rotterdam: Sense Publishers, 2013).

Index

B

C

D

E

F

R

S

T

U

V

W

Z

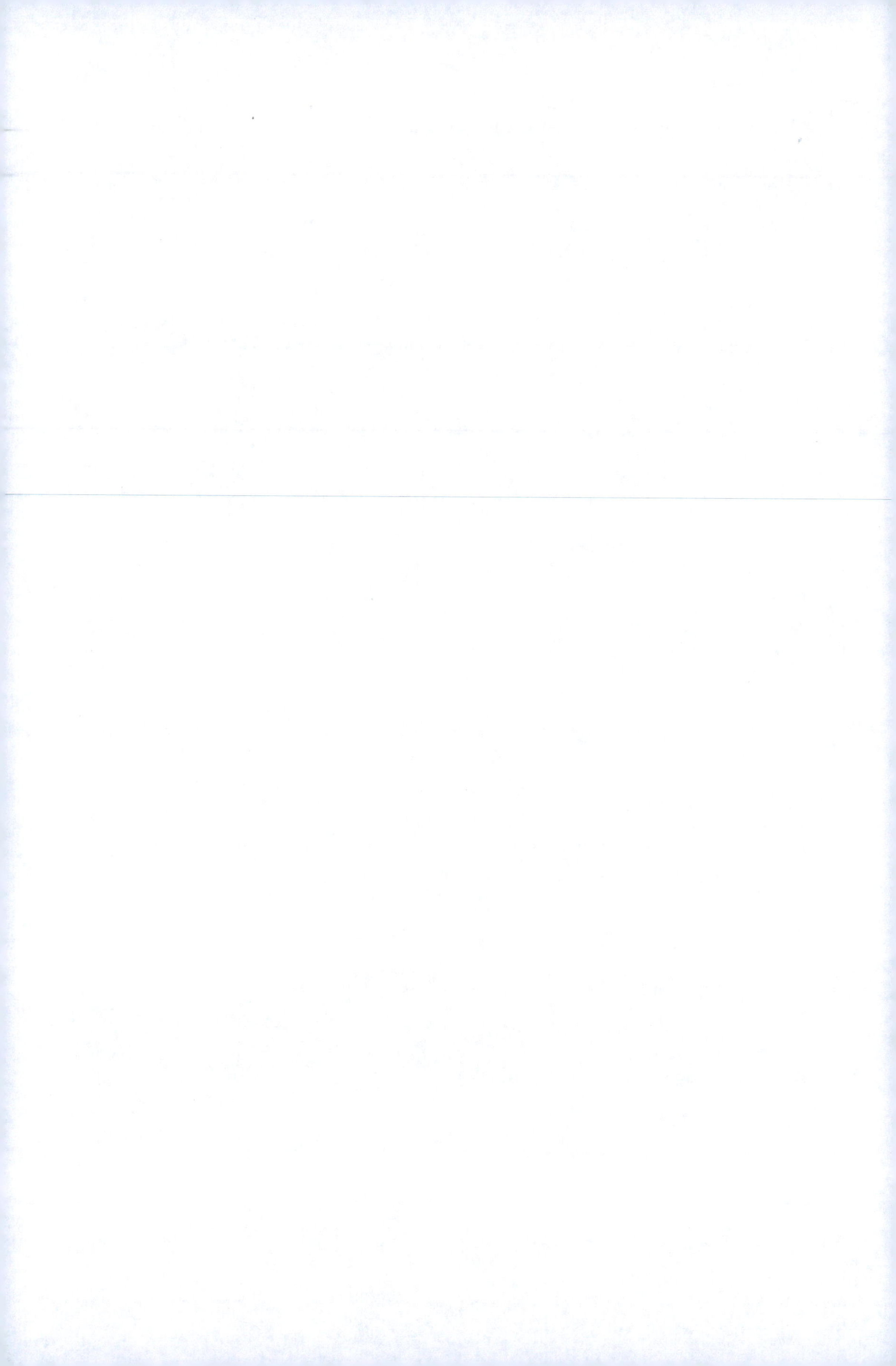